Pediatric
and Adolescent
Psychopharmacology

# Pediatric and Adolescent Psychopharmacology

## A Practical Manual for Pediatricians

Donald E. Greydanus MD
Professor, Pediatrics and Human Development, Michigan State University College of Human Medicine,
Pediatrics Program Director, Michigan State University/Kalamazoo Center for Medical Studies,
Kalamazoo, Michigan, USA

Joseph L. Calles, Jr. MD
Associate Professor, Department of Psychiatry, Michigan State University College of Human Medicine,
Director, Child and Adolescent Psychiatry, Psychiatry Program, MSU/Kalamazoo Center for Medical
Studies, Kalamazoo, Michigan, USA

Dilip R. Patel MD
Professor, Pediatrics and Human Development, Michigan State University College of Human Medicine,
Michigan State University/Kalamazoo Center for Medical Studies, Kalamazoo, Michigan, USA

Medical Illustrator: Megan M. Greydanus

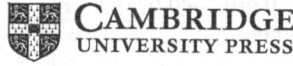

CAMBRIDGE
UNIVERSITY PRESS

# CAMBRIDGE
## UNIVERSITY PRESS

University Printing House, Cambridge CB2 8BS, United Kingdom

One Liberty Plaza, 20th Floor, New York, NY 10006, USA

477 Williamstown Road, Port Melbourne, VIC 3207, Australia

314-321, 3rd Floor, Plot 3, Splendor Forum, Jasola District Centre, New Delhi - 110025, India

103 Penang Road, #05-06/07, Visioncrest Commercial, Singapore 238467

Cambridge University Press is part of the University of Cambridge.

It furthers the University's mission by disseminating knowledge in the pursuit of education, learning and research at the highest international levels of excellence.

www.cambridge.org
Information on this title: www.cambridge.org/9780521705677

First published 2008

*A catalogue record for this publication is available from the British Library*

ISBN 978-0-521-70567-7 Paperback

..................................................................................................

Every effort has been made in preparing this book to provide accurate and up-to-date information which is in accord with accepted standards and practice at the time of publication. Although case histories are drawn from actual cases, every effort has been made to disguise the identities of the individuals involved. Nevertheless, the authors, editors and publishers can make no warranties that the information contained herein is totally free from error, not least because clinical standards are constantly changing through research and regulation. The authors, editors and publishers therefore disclaim all liability for direct or consequential damages resulting from the use of material contained in this book. Readers are strongly advised to pay careful attention to information provided by the manufacturer of any drugs or equipment that they plan to use.

# Contents

# Contributors

**Donald E. Greydanus, MD, FAAP, FSAM, FIAP (H)**
Professor of Pediatrics and Human Development
Pediatric Residency Program Director
Michigan State University College of Human Medicine
Kalamazoo Center for Medical Studies
Kalamazoo, Michigan, USA

**Joseph L. Calles, Jr. MD**
Associate Professor, Department of Psychiatry
Michigan State University College of Human Medicine
Director, Child and Adolescent Psychiatry, Psychiatry Program,
MSU/Kalamazoo Center for Medical Studies, Kalamazoo, Michigan, USA

**Dilip R. Patel, MD, FAAP, FSAM, FAACPDM, FACSM**
Professor of Pediatrics and Human Development
Michigan State University College of Human Medicine
Kalamazoo Center for Medical Studies
Kalamazoo, Michigan, USA

**Cynthia Feucht, Pharm D, BCPS**
Assistant Professor of Pharmacy Practice
Ferris State University College of Pharmacy
Michigan State University/Kalamazoo Center for Medical Studies
Kalamazoo, Michigan, USA
**(Chapters 2 and 5)**

**Helen D. Pratt, PhD**
Licensed Psychologist
Professor of Pediatric and Human Development
Michigan State University College of Human Medicine
Director of Behavioral-Developmental Pediatrics
Kalamazoo Center for Medical Studies
Kalamazoo, Michigan, USA
**(Chapter 1)**

**Artemis K. Tsitsika MD, PhD**
Pediatrics-Adolescent Medicine, Adolescent Health Unit (A.H.U.)
2nd Dpt of Pediatrics – University of Athens
"P&A Kiriakou" Children's Hospital
Athens, Greece
**(Chapter 12)**

**Eleni Tzima-Tsitsika MD**
Pediatrics-Child Development Specialist
Director of Pediatric Unit – NIMTS General Hospital
26, Plastira Str. 17121
Athens, Greece
**(Chapter 5)**

# Forewords

Children and adolescents with mental health problems commonly first present to pediatricians and primary care providers. One of the major unmet healthcare needs for children and adolescents in the USA is for the treatment of serious mental health disorders. There are far too few child and adolescent psychiatrists in the USA, and access to subspecialty expertise is often challenging. Thus, both the assessment and treatment of mental health disorders often fall to pediatricians.

*Pediatric and Adolescent Psychopharmacology*, by Greydanus, Calles, and Patel is a welcome addition to the libraries of pediatricians. This is a practical, organized text which addresses the psychopharmacologic treatment of the prominent conditions in which medications are used in children and adolescents. It is accessible, useful, and well written.

The first three chapters set the stage for pharmacologic treatment being provided in the context of comprehensive care, and addressing prescribing principles. Primary care clinicians regularly treat attention deficit/hyperactivity disorder (ADHD), writing most of the prescriptions for psychotropic medications for ADHD in the USA. ADHD is the second most common chronic illness for which pediatricians provide care. Readers will find the chapter on ADHD helpful, adding to what they know about ADHD. Pediatricians also commonly treat depression. The familiarity and comfort of pediatricians in the assessment, diagnosis, and treatment of other mental health disorders in children and adolescents are less uniform. The chapters on other disorders provide what may be new information and will be helpful to clinicians in deciding whether to broaden their scope of practice to other mental health disorders. Especially valuable are the pragmatic algorithm on the pharmacological approach to Child and Adolescent Depression and "how to use" medication, in the chapter on Disruptive Behavior and Aggressive Disorders.

This text will be of much benefit to pediatricians and all primary care clinicians.

**Christopher K. Varley, MD**
Professor
Division of Child and Adolescent Psychiatry
Department of Psychiatry and Behavioral Sciences
University of Washington School of Medicine
Seattle, WA, USA

The twenty-first century is witness to a significant number of children and adolescents presenting to pediatricians and other primary care clinicians with a wide variety of mental health problems. The offices of clinicians can be overwhelmed with children and youth that present with symptoms or diagnoses of depression, anxiety, attention deficit hyperactivity disorder, conduct disorder, psychosis, substance abuse disorders, and others. A number of medications have been developed over the past half-century or more to help improve behavior in some of these conditions. However, a shortage of child and adolescent psychiatrists in many parts of the world has left the pediatrician in the precarious position of monitoring their pediatric patients on various psychopharmacologic agents often without the help of these psychiatric consultants who are very busy themselves with new and complex patients.

*Pediatric and Adolescent Psychopharmacology* has been written to provide valuable information on these medications for pediatricians and other primary care clinicians. It is written as a guide book or "survivor's guide" for office practitioners to provide practical and very useful information on what psychopharmacologic agents are available for their pediatric patients. The authors succinctly discuss the pharmacology of these medications and include such critical information as pediatric dosages, side effects, drug interactions, which ones are FDA approved and what ages are covered by this approval, what tests must be monitored if a patient is taking them, and other data useful for such a primer of psychopharmacology. The authors are well-known experts in pediatrics, adolescent medicine, behavioral-developmental pediatrics, and child/adolescent psychiatry.

This is a very valuable book and I highly recommend it to pediatricians and other primary care clinicians who are caring for children and adolescents with mental health disorders. *Pediatric and Adolescent Psychopharmacology* will prove invaluable to help us all in providing optimal mental health care for our pediatric patients. It is a book long overdue to help in this effort!

**Renée R. Jenkins, MD FAAP**
President, American Academy of Pediatrics
Professor, Department of Pediatrics and Child Health
Howard University College of Medicine
Washington, DC, USA

# Preface

Current research suggests that 10–20% of children, adolescents, and adults suffer from mental illness, including mood disorders, anxiety disorders, attention-deficit/hyperactivity disorder, psychotic disorders, disruptive disorders (including conduct disorder), substance abuse disorders, and others. Pediatricians and other primary care clinicians are often consulted by parents for the mental health problems of their children and adolescents.

Research has occurred mainly with adults, and thus, data on children and teenagers are very limited – though now expanding. The shortage of child and adolescent psychiatrists in the world has placed considerable strain on pediatricians and primary care practitioners in helping these children and adolescents who are taking psychopharmacologic agents. The inadequate training pediatricians often receive in behavioral pediatrics and child/adolescent psychiatry is also worsened by the limited number of available books that have been written for them.

The purpose of *Pediatric and Adolescent Psychopharmacology: A Practical Manual for Pediatricians* is to provide a practical resource for pediatricians, family physicians, internists, physician assistants, nurse practitioners, and various therapists caring for millions of children and youth throughout the world, who are taking a variety of psychopharmacologic agents. Many of these medication issues are controversial and most are not officially approved for use in children or adolescents. It is essential that clinicians remain up-to-date with ever changing information and prescribing patterns.

The offices of pediatricians are flooded with patients needing, requesting, and already taking a variety of these medications. The increasing number of such medications that are being produced can place the clinician, patient, and family in a quandary about what medications, if any, to choose and how to monitor the child or adolescent already on one or several of these medications. The purpose of this book is to provide basic information and guidance on psychopharmacology in children and adolescents.

The first three chapters of this book provide an introduction to pediatric psychopharmacology, with discussions on the importance of psychological management, basics of pharmacology, and basics of prescribing psychopharmacologic agents. Then, we look at mental health disorders that pediatricians will see in their practice and that have psychopharmacologic treatments as part of their overall management plans. Thus, we provide information on medications used to manage anxiety disorders, attention-deficit/hyperactivity disorder, mood disorders, schizophrenia, autism spectrum disorders, tic disorders, and substance abuse disorders. We also provide guidance on medications used to manage children and adolescents with cognitive-adaptive disabilities and sleep disorders.

The approach we use is to provide brief comments on the definition, epidemiology, differential diagnosis, and comorbidity for each disorder. Then, we look at the psychopharmacologic medications used to manage the disorder, including classification of these medications with mechanisms of action, dosages of these medications, side-effects, and contraindications. Then, we provide information on how to use these medications and how to monitor them, noting what tests are necessary to perform while the child or adolescent is taking these psychopharmacologic agents. Each chapter ends with a limited, selected bibliography.

Much has been learned since the days of Hippocrates in regards to behavior and biology. It is the hope of the authors of this book that this information will be useful to pediatricians and primary care practitioners as they deal with children and adolescents who are taking and are in need of psychopharmacologic agents in hopes of improving the lives of our pediatric patients and successfully preparing them for adulthood.

The editors gratefully acknowledge the help of our excellent contributors in the preparation of this work: Helen D. Pratt, PhD (Chapter 1), Cynthia Feucht, Pharm D (Chapters 2 and 5), Eleni Tzima-Tsitsika, MD (Chapter 5), and Artemis K. Tsitsika, MD, PhD (Chapter 12). Finally, we also thank Deborah Russell at Cambridge University Press for her untiring faith in us and excellent expertise placing this work in print.

*Finis Coronat Opus*
Donald E. Greydanus, MD
Joseph L. Calles, Jr., MD
Dilip R. Patel, MD

# Acknowledgement

The editors gratefully acknowledge the excellent medical illustrations drawn by **Megan M. Greydanus, BFA**.

# Principles of psychological management

## Helen D. Pratt

## ■ Introduction

Physicians are often taught that pharmacological treatments are the most effective and least expensive methods of treating mental disorders. While it is true that the parents of youth who receive mental health services often have to bear a greater share of the financial burden, that burden exists because insurance companies often do not treat medical and mental illnesses with parity. Additionally, access to trained child and adolescent therapists is limited for several reasons: (a) limited numbers of clinicians are trained to deal specifically with child and adolescent issues, especially with those youth who have severe mental disorders (e.g. schizophrenia) or a combination of mental disorders and developmental disabilities, neurological disorders, or serious medical disorders; (b) many managed care panels limit the numbers of mental health clinicians they will add to their provider panels, which means that providers cannot be reimbursed for service delivery if they treat patients covered by those insurance companies; and, (c) low reimbursement rates for psychologists and social workers result in clinicians refusing to accept specific types of insurances, shifting the burden of cost to the patient's parents.

Other obstacles to referring a patient to receive psychological and psychosocial treatment include: (a) the fact that when parents and youth are in psychological distress, they want immediate relief, but psychotherapy is a time-consuming process; (b) some treatment interventions with positive outcomes often take longer to be effective than some medications do; (c) the whole family (especially parents) must devote time, energy, and effort to implementing treatment intervention; (d) youth must be transported to the treating clinician, the process of which can be disruptive to the family routine; and, (e) parents are expected to change their behaviors to support their child's treatment gains. Although parents, teachers, and some adolescents will demand pharmacological interventions first, primary care physicians should consider the use of psychological and psychosocial treatments as a first line of treatment, either alone or in combination with the prescribing of medicines.

The rationale for psychological and psychosocial interventions alone or in conjunction with pharmacotherapy includes: (a) some parents do not want their children medicated; (b) some children do not physically tolerate the medications; (c) some children reach a maximum dose on medication and can no longer be given higher doses; (d) some youth are on multiple medications and are at the point where adding more medication or increasing doses can cause serious neurological, gastrointestinal, or emotional side effects; and (e) many behavioral problems are not resolved with medication when there is an emotional component or environmental cause for the child's behavioral responses (e.g. family conflict).

This chapter presents a review of concepts and theories for the psychological management of children and adolescents with mental disorders. Topics reviewed include principles of several treatment modalities that have been shown to be effective with children and adolescents for specific disorders. The focus will be on evidence-based treatment (EBTs) because research has shown that although they are not the only effective treatments, they have consistently outperformed other care even when the youth had severe problems and were members of minority groups.

## ■ Psychotherapy

Psychotherapy is an umbrella term for the use of "talk" therapy. Clinicians practicing psychotherapy can be psychiatrists, psychologists, or social workers. These clinicians obtain special training to develop skills and competence in the delivery of specific treatment techniques based on a particular theoretical orientation. With the proper training each of them may use any or all types of therapy. The end goal for each professional is to help patients learn to change behaviors, feelings, thoughts, or habits that are causing them distress or impeding their ability to function in their personal, academic, or work lives. Clinicians generally assess the patient's needs and then, based on their theoretical orientation and their knowledge of treatment interventions, select a line of treatment designed to eliminate or minimize symptoms of emotional or behavioral dysfunction or distress.

Psychotherapy is divided into modalities (e.g. individual, group, and family) and theoretical approaches (e.g. behavioral, cognitive, eclectic, existential, interpersonal, psychoanalytic, and psychodynamic). However, in this era of evidence-based medicine, only behavioral, cognitive–behavioral, and interpersonal psychotherapies have large numbers of studies that meet the requirements to be called empirical studies.

Psychotherapy involves the therapist/clinician working to help patients understand their strengths and weaknesses, and develop strategies to minimize the negative impact of their disorder. In psychotherapy, therapists help patients identify upsetting thoughts and feelings, explore self-defeating patterns of behavior, identify difficult and potentially toxic situations and people, and learn alternative ways to handle their emotions regarding these issues. The goal is to get the patient to develop strategies to resolve or minimize their problems and to implement those strategies, then to evaluate outcomes and make adjustments to unsuccessful strategies until the goals of therapy are met. Psychotherapy is most effective with individuals who are of average to above average intelligence and who have well-developed abstract thinking and communication skills. Young children, school-age children, preadolescents, and youth who are in the early stages of developing abstract thinking (11–13 years of age) respond best to play therapy, modeling (visual examples), and art therapy.

## ■ Treatment modalities

Five forms of treatment modalities for working with youth will be presented: Individual, group, family, parent, and parent–child/adolescent. Patient diagnosis, age, preferences, family support, and financial constraints all combine to determine the manner in which therapy is delivered (modality). The principal settings are home, school, community centers, mental or medical health clinics, and private offices of the treating clinicians/therapists.

*Individual psychotherapy* is a modality wherein a single therapist delivers treatment to a single patient at a time. The type of interventions employed will be governed by the therapist's theoretical orientation and the patient's willingness to participate. The number of sessions is governed by several factors, including: (a) the patient's ability to pay; (b) insurance company's authorization; and (c) the number of sessions required to resolve a particular problem. The focus of individual therapy is on the patient's personal concerns.

*Family psychotherapy* is conducted with all or as many members as possible of a family. The therapeutic process helps identify and modify maladaptive or destructive interaction patterns, as well as foster group communication and problem-solving skills (see Table 1.1 for an example of a problem-solving technique). Techniques are delivered using interventions based on any and all of the treatment theories listed below.

*Group psychotherapy* provides patients with access to individuals with common problems where they can learn from structured interventions delivered by the clinician/therapist. In some groups, the patient's peers deliver challenges and advice under the guidance of the therapist. Most groups are homogenous and also offer a supportive environment. The groups generally meet at a specific time, in a specific place, and for a specific length of time. The groups are either open (members are allowed to attend at will and new members are allowed) or closed (a certain number of patients are allowed to participate and no new members are allowed after the first session).

*Parent–child/adolescent.* This treatment modality pairs the targeted patient with his or her parents. The presence of parents during treatment interventions is designed to provide the child with a sense of safety and a trusted role model. Parents are allowed to experience the treatment intervention with the child and sometimes model appropriate responses to reduce the child's fears or anxieties.

# ■ Theoretical approaches to psychotherapy

## Behavior therapy (BT)

The focus of this treatment modality is to teach patients and parents of patients how to increase appropriate (wanted) and decrease inappropriate (unwanted) behaviors by manipulating the patient's behavior and environment. Behavior therapy generally requires these major components: a functional analysis of the problem, contingency management, maintenance measures, generalization procedures, and self-management.

**Table 1.1** Example of a problem-solving format.

I. The first step is to examine the situation, issues, and potential impact of action
   A. Functional analysis
      1. Define the problem.
        What is the source of the problem?
      2. Who and what are involved?
      3. What aspects of the problem are controllable?
      4. What aspects are solvable?
      5. What aspects require additional help?
      6. Decide what outcome you want.
        If you don't know what you want, explore your needs.
        If there were no obstacles, what would you want in this situation?
        What would be the behavior of the others in the situation?
        What would you be doing?
        What would be the outcome?
      7. Cost–benefit analysis
        What are your options?
        What costs are involved for each option (loss relationship, fight/argument, police involvement)?
        What are the expected outcomes or consequence for each option (+ and −)?
        What kind of power does the person you are dealing with have over you?
        Does that person have the power to impact the outcome?
   B. Determine what price you are willing to pay
      1. What is your bottom line?
      2. What are you willing to give up to get what you want?
      3. Know ahead of time what you are willing to risk.
      4. Determine how you will respond if your needs are not met.
   C. Planning
      It is necessary to think this through carefully. Do not attempt problem resolution until you have carefully planned how you will approach, implement, and evaluate.
      1. Select a course of action.
      2. Design a strategy.
      3. Practice/rehearse (role play).
      4. Think about it again; repeat steps C and B.
      5. Select a day, time, and place.
      6. Be aware of your state of mind, attitudes, and confidence level: self-awareness.
      7. Be aware of the other person's state of mind, mood, receptivity, willingness to talk with you: other awareness.
      8. Pick a place where the conversation can be held in private.
        Place awareness rule: Public praise, Private criticism.

*(cont.)*

**Table 1.1** (*cont.*)

---

   D. Implementation: Do it

   E. Evaluation

     1. What was the outcome?

     2. Did you like the results?

     3. If you did not like the results, start this process again.

---

Adapted from Pratt HD, Phillips EL, Pullins P. 1987. Targeting problem behaviors in the inpatient psychiatric setting – Part I. *Behavior Management Quarterly*, 2:13–18. Note: Problem Solving Techniques are based on work by: Heppner PP, Krauskopf CJ. 1987. An information-processing approach to personal problem solving. *The Counseling Psychologist*, 15, 371–447.

*Applied behavior analysis* (ABA) is the foundation of behavior therapy. Principles of reinforcement, punishment, and schedules of reinforcement/punishment are important procedures in this theory. Therapists, teachers, and parents can be taught to use the principles of ABA to teach new behaviors (wanted behaviors), eliminate unwanted behaviors, and develop programs of treatment to address most behavioral problems.

*Behavior modification* (BMod) is the term used to label the process of changing the behavior of the individual. Behavior modification encompasses the principles of ABA and uses the techniques listed below in interventions designed to change behavior. Parents and teachers are often taught BMod techniques for managing the behavior of youth in the home and students in the classroom. *Change agent* is the term used to describe parents and teachers who have been trained in BMod. Used correctly, BMod is a very powerful technique. As with all forms of therapy, incorrect application can produce unwanted results.

*Functional analysis* is a process employed to identify what is causing and maintaining or preventing specific targeted behaviors. During a functional analysis of the problem several steps are employed: (1) identification of problem behavior; (2) determining the antecedents, consequences and maintaining variables controlling the behavior; (3) selecting or targeting behavior to be changed; (4) identifying and selecting potential rewards and punishers; (5) goal setting and developing specific criteria for determining when goals are met; (6) identifying consequences (rewards and punishers); (7) fading or thinning of consequence to maintain gains; and (8) planning for the termination of the program.

*Contingency management* involves the development of a detailed reward and punishment system wherein techniques such as token economies, timeouts, over correction, and response cost might be employed. These interventions allow patients to learn new target behaviors. Another intervention is called shaping, which allows the patient to learn a new behavior in small parts, starting with an existing positive or appropriate behavior. Once new or targeted responses are learned via a series of successive approximations, the individual is then required to make responses that are more complex until the target behavioral response is reliably performed under specific stimulus conditions. The purpose of using this system is to increase adaptive, prosocial, and appropriate behaviors and eliminate or reduce maladaptive or inappropriate behaviors in specific settings.

*Self-management* requires that the individual learns self-observation/monitoring, self-analysis, self-instruction, and self-evaluation, as well as task and time management, and problem-solving strategies/skills. Individuals are taught to use behavioral techniques to increase their awareness and control of their own behaviors.

*Systematic desensitization* involves slowly introducing a fear- or anxiety-provoking stimulus to the child or adolescent until that stimulus no longer elicits a fearful or anxious response in the individual. Components can include exposure, graduated exposure, modeling (videos, tapes, role plays), and flooding (exposure to the negative stimulus, full force, until it no longer elicits a negative response). Variations in the actual format of the techniques are described in the literature.

## Family systems theory

This theory is based on the premise that family dynamics and communications affect the function of family members. By helping members modify problem dynamics within the family, positive changes can be made to improve the family's ability to be a positive environment for its members. The focus is on examination of the interpersonal and group dynamics of the family. Therapists help the family examine its communication process, behaviors, values, beliefs, and practices. Interventions from BT, CBT (see below), psychoanalysis, and social psychology are adapted to address the family issues and problems. The therapist works with family members individually and collectively to deal with the relationships of parent–parent, parent(s)–child, child–parent(s), child–child, child–all family members, and parent(s)–children. Issues such as triangulation (two family members joining forces to counter another family member; usually parent–child against another parent or two parents against a child), conflict management, anger management, self-control, child management, and interpersonal relationship management are addressed.

## Cognitive–behavioral therapy (CBT)

This is a structured and directive method of therapy designed to help youth work on immediate issues and change their maladaptive behaviors. Cognitive–behavioral therapy combines components of psychotherapy, behavior therapy, and social psychology, and includes stress management, relaxation training, social skills training, support groups, parent training, teacher training, and peer mediation. These interventions are selectively used to help people rethink and restructure how they feel and think about their actions, with the end goal of helping to initiate behavior change. Cognitive–behavioral therapy uses the Socratic Method to help adolescents think through their problems and employs induction to help challenge assumptions with rational thinking and factual information. Youth learn how to think through tasks and organize work, as well as engage in problem solving, planning, and time management.

*Cognitive restructuring* is designed to help the adolescent detect, recognize, and challenge irrational or highly negative beliefs, guilt, hopelessness, and thoughts of worthlessness. The therapist helps the individual follow a set of steps based on a problem-solving model to determine the actual outcome of the adolescent's current beliefs and to generate possible reactions and solutions to the worst case scenarios. The adolescent then practices the solutions with the therapist until mastery is achieved, then tries out the solutions one at a time in the real world. Therapy is designed to be time limited.

## Social learning theory

This theory holds that individuals can be taught to interact with other people in a socially appropriate manner. Training involves techniques from BT and social psychology.

*Social skills training* is often used as a component of treatment packages, as a means of teaching or increasing a child's prosocial behavior such as waiting for a turn, sharing toys, asking for help, responding appropriately to teasing, effectively making friends, and imitating the proper role models. Models of appropriate and inappropriate social behavior are presented to the child. The models (via videos or in vivo) are then discussed as to why such behavior is acceptable, and the trainer then explains why the inappropriate models are not okay. Learners then practice and receive corrective feedback. Trainers then use contingency management techniques and group activities to help learners make appropriate comments. This process is designed to help the participants learn to view their own personal behavior and how that behavior affects others; additionally participants are encouraged to develop new ways to respond when feeling angry, pushed, frustrated, scared, afraid, sad, etc.

*Support groups* provide individuals with common concerns a way to come together to learn and share their issues, experiences, strengths, weaknesses, frustrations, and successes. They may also be a resource for referrals to qualified specialists, for information about what works, as well as a forum for parents to discuss their hopes for themselves and their children. Support groups are useful with adults, teens, and children. Such groups can be organized around any supportive person, such as a parent, teen, or teacher, and can include peer mediation groups. Support groups can be local, regional, state, and national.

*Parenting training* is designed to help parents improve their parenting effectiveness and ultimately the quality of life for their whole family. Interventions are used to teach parents about child development, child management, contingency management, stress management, and relaxation techniques. They provide parents with tools and techniques for managing their child's behavior and how to teach their children coping skills for handling their particular disorder.

Specific issues addressed during training include identifying specific information on why children misbehave, how to pay attention (positive attending and ignoring), how to increase compliance and independent play, token economies, punishment (time out, response cost), and anticipating problems such as how to manage children in public places. Additionally parents are taught techniques for rewarding positive school behaviors, and how to handle future behavior problems. Follow-up sessions are conducted to troubleshoot and support parents, combined with follow-up parent meetings. This form of therapy works best with parents who are mentally healthy, have a healthy marriage, and share similar beliefs about how children should be raised. The current treatment programs for parent training can be adjusted to meet the needs of parents who have limited intellectual functioning or are undergoing concurrent individual psychotherapy. Settings for treatment include the therapist's private office, community centers, community mental and medical health settings, schools, etc. Social skills activity groups are often held concurrently with parent training/support groups.

*Teacher training* is designed to help teachers improve their classroom management skills and to support the therapeutic gains their students made while in treatment. Teachers are most effective when they involve children by teaching them self-management techniques (such as recording their own appropriate or inappropriate behaviors), combined with teacher observation and feedback on the accuracy of the child's self-monitoring recordings. Contingency management techniques that include individual, team, and class contingencies are the most effective. Teacher classroom management also improves when their intervention programs provide a clear, consistent system for translating teacher reports into consequences at home.

*Peer mediation* programs in schools access a wider range of youth than do traditional treatment programs. They overcome obstacles to treatment such as lack of access, financial constraints, refusal of parents to participate, and adolescent resistance to psychotherapy. Student-mediated conflict resolution programs consist of a trained team of older youth to help peers solve conflicts and have occurred in schools and private offices. Successful programs must have administrative support and commitment to the goals and practices of the program by the majority of teachers and parents. The inclusion of parents and high-risk students as trained mediators improves the overall environment.

## Biofeedback

Biofeedback involves the use of equipment that allows the child or adolescent to become aware of his or her physiological responses to stimuli. For example, an electrode is attached to the child's finger to monitor his or her skin moisture (galvanic skin response). The child or adolescent sees a visual image or hears a sound that changes with varying levels of moisture in the child/adolescent's finger. The individual is then taught to alter his or her thoughts, relaxing the tension in his or her muscles, and/or by controlling his or her breathing.

## Interpersonal psychosocial therapy (IPT)

Interpersonal psychosocial therapy focuses on helping youth address behavior symptoms and interpersonal interactions. The premise is that each individual's personality is the culmination of recurrent patterns of interpersonal interactions. The way the individual communicates is a major part of those interactions and plays a major role in the development and sequelae of adolescent depression. These theorists believe that IPT is especially relevant to working with adolescents, because during this developmental phase youth are expanding their social interaction worlds and struggle to initiate and maintain social relationships with peers and significant others. Treatment focuses on helping individuals process their feeling of loss by helping them: (a) effectively mourn perceived or real losses; (b) reestablish interests in activities, people, life; (c) manage the complexities of interpersonal and intimate relationships; (d) settle interpersonal disputes; (e) prepare for role transitions; (f) recognize and deal with their own interpersonal deficits; (g) deal with the dynamics of a single-parent family (if applicable); and (h) recognize disputes and engage in activities that allow them to develop plans of action to modify their communications and expectations.

# ■ Psychosocial treatments for selected child and adolescent mental disorders

## Anxiety disorders

Behavioral treatments for anxiety disorders include CBT and BT (graduated exposure, systematic desensitization, modeling, implosion, flooding, etc.). A list of specific disorders of anxiety and their related behavioral treatments are included in Table 1.2.

## Attention deficit/hyperactivity disorder (ADHD)

The National Institute of Mental Health reports that based on their research, combined BT and medication therapy was more effective for specific groups of children and adolescents diagnosed with ADHD; this included children with parent-defined comorbid anxiety disorders and particularly those with overlapping disruptive disorder. Effective bio-psychosocial treatment packages for treating ADHD in children and adolescents should include CBT, BT, social-skills training, and self-management training, all of which can be delivered with individuals and groups. Peer mediation (in schools), support groups (one for parents and one for youth), parenting training, and teacher training are also useful components.

**Table 1.2** Evidence-based treatments for anxiety disorders.

| Type of fear | Treatment formats | Treatment interventions |
|---|---|---|
| *Specific fears* | | |
| Blood | Individual | Relaxation |
| | | Systematic desensitization |
| Buses | Individual | Exposure |
| Dogs | Individual | Exposure |
| | Group | Modeling (with either neutral or positive context) |
| | | Modeling (with either multiple or single filmed models) |
| | | Modeling with mother as model |
| Choking | Individual | Reinforced practice |
| Dark | Individual | Exposure |
| | | Graduated exposure |
| | | In vivo exposure |
| Dental | Individual | Participant modeling |
| | | Coping model – video modeling |
| Heights | Individual | Relaxation |
| | | Systematic desensitization |
| Illness | Individual | Imaginal exposure |
| Injections | Individual | Modeling film |
| Medical procedures | Individual | Modeling alone |
| | | Modeling with mother present |
| | | Puppet modeling |
| Mixed phobias | Individual with child with parent present | Exposure |
| Public speaking | Group | Imaginal exposure |
| Separation Illness | Individual | Imaginal exposure |
| Snakes | Group | Child modeling |
| | Individual | Live modeling with guided participation |
| | | Symbolic modeling contact |
| | | Desensitization systematic |
| | | Desensitization live modeling |
| | | Vicarious desensitization |
| Social isolation | Group | Coaching with video |
| | | Modeling plus coaching with video |

**Table 1.2** (*cont.*)

| Type of fear | Treatment formats | Treatment interventions |
|---|---|---|
| Spider phobia | Individual | Modeling with video |
| | | Modeling with video plus Reinforcement |
| | | In Vivo exposure |
| | | Modeling plus exposure to analog – delayed or immediate or spaced |
| | | Modeling plus exposure either delayed, immediate, spaced |
| Surgery in hospital | Individual | Modeling with slide show |
| Swimming | Individual | Participation |
| | | Modeling |
| Talking to adults | Parent–child | Participant modeling with mother as model |
| Travel | Individual | Imaginal exposure |
| *Anxieties* | | |
| Night-time fears | Individual | Emotive imagery |
| High anxiety | Individual | Relaxation plus exposure |
| Obsessive-compulsive disorder | Individual Group family | Graded exposure, Exposure and response prevention (ERP) |
| | | Response prevention |
| | | Cognitive techniques |
| | | Family therapy/involvement. Follow-up sessions |
| Panic attacks | Individual group | Behavioral therapy (implosion, flooding, systematic desensitization) including CBT have been shown to be effective in eliminating or reducing panic attacks |
| Separation Anxiety | Parent–child Individual | CBT including relaxation techniques, positive self-statements, token program aimed at rewarding nonfearful responses, and cognitive control of fearful thoughts |

(*cont.*)

**Table 1.2** (*cont.*)

| Type of fear | Treatment formats | Treatment interventions |
|---|---|---|
| Social anxiety | Group Individual | Systematic desensitization CBT |
| Social phobia | Group Individual | CBT that involves treatments like systematic desensitization, implosion and flooding are very effective forms of psychotherapy |
| Specific phobia | Group Individual | CBT that involves treatments like systematic desensitization, implosion and flooding are very effective forms of psychotherapy. |
| Test anxiety | Group Individual | Exposure plus relaxation Group direct desensitization Imaginal desensitization Systematic desensitization Systematic desensitization plus relaxation Group vicarious desensitization |
| Trauma | Individual | Imaginal flooding |
| Post traumatic stress disorder | | CBT taught methods of overcoming anxiety or depression and modifying undesirable behaviors such as avoidance of reminders of the traumatic event. |

Adapted from Chorpita BF, Southam-Gero MA. 2006. Fears and anxieties. In Marsh EJ, Barkley RA (Eds.) *Treatment of Childhood Disorders 3rd edn.*, pp. 314–25. New York: Guilford Press.

## Autistic spectrum disorders (ASD)

There is no single best treatment package for all children with ASD. However, most specialists agree that early intervention is important, and that individuals with ASD respond well to programs that include: (a) a sustained, highly structured environment that employs specialized, intensive interventions that are based on principles of ABA; (b) parent training that is educative and supportive; (c) a curriculum that focuses on the social and communication domains; (d) instruction that is systematic, with goals and objectives that are tailored to the unique developmental, ethnic, and cultural needs of the individual and family; and (e) an emphasis on eventual generalization of therapeutic gains. A second area of agreement is the need to provide an intensive intervention program that emphasizes the generalization (across a variety of settings) of positive behaviors and skills. When instituted with the collaboration of parents, positive outcomes are typically obtained. Other essential therapies include social skills training, speech/language therapy, occupational therapy, and physical therapy when relevant to the child's needs. Therapy should also be provided to parents and siblings via support groups.

## Cognitive-adaptive disabilities

Mental retardation (MR) is a nonspecific term for youth who have obtained below normal intellectual quotients on standardized tests and also have deficits in functioning two or more standard deviations below the mean on measures of activities of living. The principles of psychiatric treatment are the same as for persons without MR, but modification of techniques may be necessary according to the individual patient's level of cognitive development, especially communication skills. Youth with medical illnesses, physical disabilities, and impaired cognitive functioning will benefit most from a coordinated and comprehensive treatment program.

Behavior therapy is the most effective form of treatment with youth with moderate to severe mental retardation. These youth may retain some level of abstract thinking abilities and can therefore benefit from "talk therapies;" however, treatment interventions must be modified to account for their limited ability to understand and express their thoughts and feelings. The addition of visual aids and prompts to promote learning and understanding can be useful in therapy. Treatment techniques that are focused on current reality, directive and structured are more effective. Those youth who have comorbid mood disorders will need to have treatment modified to meet their individual needs.

Individuals with severe MR are better treated with BT with a focus on techniques from ABA. Parents of adolescents and young adults diagnosed with MR may need extra help in coming to terms with emergent sexuality. The youth will need to engage in transitional activities, to prepare those who are candidates for independent living to emotionally separate and prepare for moving to out-of-family living in their communities.

## Depression in childhood

According to the National Institutes of Mental health, short term (10–20 week) talk therapy is effective in treating those individuals who can benefit from this form of therapy. CBT, BT, and IPT are all effective treatments for treating youth diagnosed with depression. In general, youth with severe depressive illnesses, those who have recurrent depression or who are suicidal, will require pharmacotherapy combined with psychotherapy. Under special circumstances, electroconvulsive therapy (ECT) may be indicated.

## Disruptive behavior disorders (DBD)

Youth who are aggressive will require a combination of several treatment interventions. They will need to learn how to recognize, assess, avoid, or prevent dangerous situations. They will also need to learn better social skills and self-control and self-management skills. Cognitive–behavioral therapy, BT, and IPT are effective treatment interventions. Settings include home, school, residential treatment centers, and private therapist's offices. The adults in their environments must provide them with a structured setting where they feel safe, supported, and have opportunities to engage in conflict management and negotiation skills. Additionally, it is easier for these youth to engage in prosocial behavior if their peers buy into the concept of peer mediation and are willing to adhere to the mediated solutions to conflict.

*Conduct disorders* (CD) represent a constellation of anti-social behaviors. Behavioral treatment for youth diagnosed with CD is delivered via individual and group therapy, with expectations for behavior and consequences for noncompliance clearly spelled out and administered. Treatment packages for therapy with these youth contain modules on problem-solving, cognitive restructuring, conflict negotiation, self-assessment, self-control, and self-management. Youth learn prosocial behavior (via modeling and direct reinforcement), such as empathy, sympathy, altruism, assertiveness (versus aggressiveness), politeness, responsibility, trustworthiness, and dependability. Youth also learn how to recognize their mistakes and how to make restitution without coercion (e.g., saying "I'm sorry"). Activities involving structured tasks (such as games, academic activities, and story telling) help these youth apply the lesson they learn in therapy to real-life situations in a supervised situation. This outpatient therapy is not effective unless the parents and teachers learn behavior management skills (as in BT) and become effective change agents. Their families must also participate in family therapy to help them make corresponding changes at home that will support the youth's treatment gains.

Youth with conduct disorders who do not respond to outpatient therapy may benefit from being placed in a residential facility. Effective residential treatment programs, for youth with serious conduct problems and comorbid affective disorders, generally combine the theories of BT, CBT, and multisystemic family therapy to design their programs and develop the corresponding interventions. The focus is on teaching youth social skills from a standardized skills curriculum. Token-economies are used to motivate prosocial behaviors and minimize antisocial behavior. Youth live at the facilities for about one year and are provided with a structured environment where each person has responsibilities (e.g. cooking, cleaning, laundry, yard work, etc.); privileges, family contact, and home visits are earned. School attendance (generally on-site) is required, and participation in extracurricular activities (sports, recreational/leisure) is strongly encouraged. Most programs allow youth to participate in some form of self-governance. School-based interventions are usually based on the same theories, but only include peer mediation, parent and teacher training, conflict negotiation, and self-management techniques.

*Oppositional defiant disorder* (ODD) is a constellation of behaviors that describe youth who are often noncompliant and defiant. Youth diagnosed with ODD will also need intensive treatment interventions, which include some version of those listed above, especially parent training. Young children who exhibit these symptoms will generally benefit from having their parents become effective change agents. Adolescents will need a combination of individual therapy and group therapy based on BT and CBT. Oppositional defiant disorder is the least serious of the disruptive behavior disorders.

## Elimination disorders

Youth in the USA are expected to have full control of their bowel and bladder by age 2.5 years, but definitely by the time youth enter elementary school. Children who are ready for toilet training usually have conscious control over their bladders, with increasingly longer periods (several hours) of time where the diaper is dry, awareness of the need to void, and the ability to understand and follow simple instructions. Children with motor and developmental delays, autism, and mental retardation may not learn toileting skills by these ages, but can benefit from modified versions of behavior therapy for toilet training.

*Encopresis* involves constipation, withholding of stool, and fecal soiling. After all medical causes and organic etiologies for chronic constipation are ruled out, medical and behavioral treatments can begin. It is essential that parents understand that treatment for constipation can take many months of continued efforts. Parents must also be assured that their child is not at fault for soiling. Treatment involves a combined approach of medical and behavioral interventions. The first step is the complete evacuation of the bowels (disimpaction); next the focus is on prevention of re-accumulation of the stool by using stool softeners and laxatives (the colon is thus able to return to normal caliber and tone). The next step is to use biofeedback to teach the patient to learn how to know when he or she needs to defecate, and to be able to control the timing of that behavior. Biofeedback with a balloon probe inserted into the patient's anus teaches the patient to contract and constrict, and relax anal muscles. The child is presented with visual images designed to teach voluntary squeeze control of the anal sphincter and recognize the associated physiological sensations. Once these goals are accomplished the process continues with a gradual weaning of the laxative regimen and the institution of a toilet training program. The next step is to implement toilet training as described below.

*Enuresis* refers to the behavior of wetting one's bed at night or wetting one's underpants during the day. It is either *primary* (the child has never attained control) or *secondary* (the person was once potty trained, but wetting has recurred). All toilet training programs are designed to motivate and reward compliance with toilet training activities. Behavioral therapy treatments include an enuresis alarm bell (dry pants/underwear) and/or alarm pad (dry bed). The sound of the alarm is a part of an operant conditioning technique and has the highest rates of success in nocturnal enuresis. The sound of the bell occurs when dampness is detected in the underwear or on the bed pad. The alarm wakes the child up, causing the muscles in the bladder to contract, stopping the flow of urine. The basic components include: (a) increased fluid intake (to increase bladder capacity); (b) regularly scheduled toilet times; (c) positive reinforcement for correct elimination (verbal statements, tokens, stickers); (d) overcorrection for accidents (i.e. the youth is required to change bed, underwear, and wash soiled laundry) (the level of involvement in this process is determined by the age and developmental level of the child/adolescent); (e) consistent and systematic parent responses to alarms and the youth's request to toilet; and (f) the youth's motivation to participate voluntarily in the process. This technique is labor and time intensive but has been successfully modified to work even in special needs populations.

## Schizophrenia in childhood and adolescence

Once the child or adolescent with schizophrenia has been stabilized on antipsychotic medications (that deal with certain aspects of schizophrenia, such as difficulty with communication, motivation, self-care, work, and establishing and maintaining relationships with others), they can benefit from CBT, IPT, and BT to help them learn and use coping mechanisms to address these problems. Because social skills become so impaired during an episode of psychosis or during the decompensation phase, these youth will benefit from social skills and coping skills interventions.

## Substance abuse in adolescents

Psychotherapy is an integral part of treatment for substance abuse and the frequent accompanying mental disorders. Treatment is often multi-disciplinary in approach and may include psychiatric hospitalization, residential placement, or outpatient therapy to receive family education, CBT, BT, IPT, self-help groups, manualized treatments, drug court, family court services, and surveillance. These programs have been show to be effective in decreasing rates of adolescent substance use and criminal behavior; however, relapse rates are high.

# ■ Psychosocial treatments for selected child and adolescent behavioral disorders

## Self injury

Prevention of the self-injurious behavior is the primary focus of treatment. A secondary focus is to teach alternative responses. Applied behavior analysis in particular (differential reinforcement of other behaviors [DRO], differential reinforcement of intervals [DRI] plus interruption [DRI-I]) were effective at reducing or eliminating serious self-injury in youth diagnosed with mental retardation or autism. Some behavioral techniques for extremely severe self-injurious behavior (e.g. electrical shocks) have been controversial. Issues with frustration, anger, and self-stimulation are all factors that must be addressed when designing treatment (see Table 1.3 for resources for specific treatments).

## Sleep disorders

Most sleeping problems for children and youth are the result of no bedtime routine or inconsistent parental command and consequences for going to bed and going to sleep. Small children find that they can get parental attention if they keep getting out of bed and demand things (asking for things like a drink or to go to the toilet) or by telling their parents they "love" them. Many homes have competing activities that draw children into wanting to stay up. It is important to establish a clear, consistent, relaxing bedtime routine for small children to teach good sleep hygiene. For example, the bedtime routine begins at 7:00 p.m. with the youth in the bed at 8:00 and asleep by 8:15. This means that the parents must start the process at 7:00 p.m. with announcing it is time to get ready for bed, turning off the television, eliminating all other distractions, give or have one take a bath/shower, get into sleeping clothes, brush teeth, toilet, read story, hug/cuddle, toilet, get a drink of water, get in bed, turn lights out (leave night light for youth who are afraid of dark), say good night, and go to sleep.

Adolescents too have sleep problems but most are also related to bedtime routines that are incompatible with going to sleep. Most adolescents with sleep problems are often distracted by televisions, video games, and telephone conversations when it is time to go to sleep. They then stay awake late or all night, have problems getting up in the morning and want to sleep all day. This can result in learning problems, lost school days, and lack of school attendance. The same routines for sleep hygiene are as important for adolescents as for young children.

Youth who are unable to sleep because they are taking medications that interfere with sleep patterns will need to be reevaluated by their physicians and then start a sleep hygiene program to restore their ability to go to sleep and remain asleep.

Treatment of sleep walking often involves making sure that the patient establishes a bedtime routine, is getting adequate sleep, and the home is safe. Some interventions require alarms to alert parents, but not startle the

**Table 1.3** Additional resources for evidence-based psychosocial treatment of emotional, behavioral, and mental disorders of childhood.

General

Note: This is an example of manualized treatment:

Bloomquist ML. 2006. *Skills Training for Children with Behavior Problems: A Parent and Practitioner Guidebook, Rev. edn.* New York: Guilford Press.

Reinecke MA, Dattilio FM, Freeman A. 1996. *Cognitive Therapy with Children and Adolescents: A Casebook for Clinical Practice.* New York: Guilford Press.

Robin A, Foster SL. 1989. *Negotiating Parent-Adolescent Conflict: A Behavioral-Family Systems Approach.* New York: Guilford Press.

Weiner JM. 1997. *Textbook of Child and Adolescent Psychiatry, 2nd edn.* Washington, DC: American Psychiatric Press.

Aggressive behavior

Note: This is an example of manualized treatment:

Goldstein AP, Glick B, Reiner S, Zimmerman D Coultry TM. 1987. *Aggression Replacement Training: A Comprehensive Intervention for Aggressive Youth.* Champaign, IL: Research Press.

*Note: This is an example of manualized treatment:*

Goldstein AP, Palumbo J, Striepling S, Voutsinas AM. 1995. *Break it Up: A Teacher's Guide to Managing Student Aggression.* Champaign, IL: Research Press.

Green RW, Ablon JS. 2006. *Treating Explosive Kids: The Collaborative Problem-solving Approach.* New York: Guilford Press.

Putallaz M, Bierman KL (Eds.) 2004. *Aggression, Antisocial Behavior, and Violence among Girls: A Developmental Perspective.* New York: Guilford Press.

Anxiety disorders

Cohen JA, Mannarion AP, Deblinger E. 2006. *Treating Trauma and Traumatic Grief in Children and Adolescents.* New York: Guilford Press.

Attention deficit/hyperactivity disorder (ADHD)

Barkley RA. 2000. *Taking Charge of ADHD: the Complete, Authoritative Guide for Parents.* New York: Guilford Press.

Autism

Siegel B. 1996. *The World of the Autistic Child: Understanding and Treating Autistic Spectrum Disorders.* New York: Oxford University Press.

Conduct disorders

Bloomquist ML, Schnell S. 2002. *Helping Children with Aggressive and Conduct Problems: Best Practices for Intervention.* New York: Guilford Press.

Noncompliance/ Oppositional behavior

McMahon RJ, Forehand RL. 2003. *Helping the Noncompliant Child: Family-based Treatment for Oppositional Behavior, 2nd edn.* New York: Guilford Press.

patient. Parents are advised to establish a bedtime routine and consistently implement that routine. Interventions include contingency management to gain compliance with going to and staying in bed. Interventions might look like this: If bed time is at 8:00, start getting ready for bed at 7:00; announce it is time to get ready for bed. Then give baths (parents should participate in this process at varying levels that are dictated by the age of the child and safety precautions). Next, have children put on sleeping clothes and gather in a central spot. Parents then can do story time with soothing and fun stories with all children in the home. Next have each child go to his or her respective sleeping place and get into bed. Make sure things like toileting, tooth brushing, drinks of water, and hugs are all done. Dim or turn out the lights.

## Conclusion

Psychosocial treatments for emotional, behavioral, and mental disorders can be very effective and sufficient in resolving problems. Emotional problems resulting from medical disorders can also be effectively addressed with psychosocial treatments. However, in the case of severe or recurring emotional, behavioral, and mental disorders, a combination of pharmacotherapy and psychotherapy increase the positive effects of treatment. Youth should receive a comprehensive medical evaluation prior to being referred for psychosocial treatment. When referring patients for psychotherapy, it is important to remember to tell them and their parents that the process for accessing treatment, getting evaluated for treatment, and the treatment process is often lengthy. Treatments are also labor intensive for parents, patients, and teachers. But the outcome of such treatment is that youth may actually learn to implement effective techniques to help themselves manage future problems.

SELECTED BIBLIOGRAPHY

Azrin NH, Foxx RM. 1971. A rapid method of toilet training the institutionalized retarded. *J. Appl. Behav. Analysis*, 4:89–99.

Barkley RA (Ed.) 1998. *Attention-Deficit Hyperactivity Disorder: A Handbook for Diagnosis and Treatment, 2nd edn*. New York: Guilford Press, pp. 458–90.

Buchanan A, Claydon G. 1992. *Children who Soil: Assessment and Treatment*. Chichester: John Wiley and Sons.

Compton SN, Nelson AH, March JS. 2000. Social phobia and separation anxiety symptoms in community and clinical samples of children and adolescents. *J. Am. Acad. Child Adolesc. Psychiatry*, 39(8):1040–6.

Croffie JMB, Fitzgerald JF. 1996. Idiopathic constipation. In Walker WA, Durie RR, Hamilton JR, Walker-Smith JA, Watkins JB (Eds.) *Pediatric Gastrointestinal Disease, 2nd edn.* St Louis: Mosby Yearbook, pp. 984–97.

Henggeler SW, Halliday-Boykins CA, Cunningham PB, Randall J, Shapiro B, Chapman JE. 2006. Juvenile drug court: enhancing outcomes by integrating evidence-based treatments. *J. Consult. Clin. Psychol.*, 74(1):42–54.

Hillman J. 2006. Supporting and treating families with children on the autistic spectrum: the unique role of the generalist psychologist. *Psychotherapy: Theory, Research, Practice, Training*, 43(3):349–58.

Jensen PS, Hinshaw SP, Kraemer HC, et al. 2001. ADHD comorbidity findings from the MTA study: comparing comorbid subgroups. *J. Am. Acad. Child Adolesc. Psychiatry*, 40:147–58.

Kazdin, AE, Weisz JR. 2003. *Evidence-Based Psychotherapies for Children and Adults.* New York: Guilford Press.

Lewin AB, Storch, EA, Adkins JW, et al. 2005. Update and review of pediatric obsessive-compulsive disorder. *Psychiatr. Ann.*, 35(9):745–53.

Malott RW, Malott, ME, Trojan, EA. 2000. *Elementary Principles of Behavior, 4th edn.* Upper Saddle River, NJ: Prentice Hall.

Marsh EJ, Barkley RA (Eds.) 1998. *Treatment of Childhood Disorders, 3rd edn.* New York: Guilford Press, pp. 314–25.

McNeil DW, Zvolensky MJ. 2000. Systematic desensitization. In Kazdin, AE. (Ed.) *Encyclopedia of Psychology*, 7:533–5.

Mufson L, Dorta KP. 2003. Interpersonal psychotherapy for depressed adolescents. In Kazdin AE, Weisz JR (Eds.) *Evidence-Based Psychotherapies for Children and Adults.* New York: Guilford Press, pp. 148–64.

National Association of Cognitive-Behavioral Therapists (NACBT). 2006. *What is Cognitive-Behavior Therapy?* Bethesda, MD: NACBT. Available at: http://www.nacbt.org/whatiscbt.htm

National Institute of Mental Health (NIMH). 1999. *Facts about Obsessive-Compulsive Disorder.* Bethesda, MD. Publication OM-99 4154 (Revised). Available at: http://www.nimh.nih.gov/publicat/ocdfacts.cfm

National Institute of Mental Health (NIMH). 2000. *Child and Adolescent Bipolar Disorder: An Update from the National Institute of Mental Health.* Bethesda, MD. NIH Publication No. 00–4778. Available at: http://www.nimh.nih.gov/publicat/bipolarupdate.cfm

National Institute of Mental Health. 2000. *Depression in Children and Adolescents.* Bethesda, MD NIMH. NIH Publication No. 00–4744. Available at: http://www.nimh.nih.gov/publicat/depchildresfact.cfm

National Institute of Mental Health (NIMH). 2001. *Attention Deficit Hyperactivity Disorder.* Bethesda, MD: NIMH. Publication No. 01–4589. Available at: http://www.nimh.nih.gov/publicat/helpchild.cfm

National Institute of Mental Health (NIMH). 2006. *Autism Spectrum Disorders (Pervasive Developmental Disorders)*. Bethesda, MD: NIMH. Available at: http://www.nimh.nih.gov/healthinformation/autismmenu.cfm

National Institute of Mental Health (NIMH), National Institutes of Health (NIH) U.S. Department of Health and Human Services. 2006. *Schizophrenia*. Bethesda, MD. Available at: http://www.nimh.nih.gov/publicat/schizoph.cfm#treatment

Patel DR, Pratt HD. 1999. Encopresis. *Indian J. Pediatr.*, 66(3):439–46.

Pfiffner LJ, Calzada E, McBurnett K. 2000. Interventions to enhance social competence. *Child Adolesc. Psychiatr. Clin. N. Am.*, 9(3):689–709.

Szymanski L. 1999. Practice parameters for the assessment and treatment of children, adolescents, and adults with mental retardation and comorbid mental disorders. *J. Am. Acad. Child Adolesc. Psychiatry*, 38(2):5S–31S.

Weiner JM. 1997. *Textbook of Child and Adolescent Psychiatry, 2nd edn*. Washington, DC: American Psychiatric Press.

Weisz JR, Jensen-Doss A, Hawley KM. 2006. Evidence-based youth psychotherapies versus usual clinical care: a meta-analysis of direct comparisons. *Am. Psychologist*, 61(7):671–89.

Wolfe DA, Mash EJ (Eds.) 2006. *Behavioral and Emotional Disorders in Adolescence: Nature, Assessment, and Treatment*. New York: Guilford Press.

Wolpe J. 1958. *Psychotherapy by Reciprocal Inhibition*. Stanford, CA: Stanford University Press.

# The basics of pharmacology and neurotransmission

## Dilip R. Patel and Cynthia Feucht

This chapter reviews basic concepts of pharmacology and neurotransmission applicable to psychotherapeutic agents used for the treatment of mental disorders of children and adolescents. An understanding of the basic principles of pharmacokinetics and pharmacodynamics of drugs is important in the appropriate therapeutic use of various drugs.

In simple terms the effects of the body on the drug once it has entered the body has been referred to as *pharmacokinetics*, and it aims to provide a quantitative assessment of the main processes involved in the biodisposition of the drug which include absorption, distribution, metabolism, and elimination. On the other hand, *pharmacodynamics* concerns itself with the effects of the drug on the body and the main processes involved are the action of the drug on specific sites, especially the receptors.

## ■ Pharmacokinetics

### Absorption

A drug can be administered via various routes and the specific route chosen largely depends upon the urgency to achieve the desired effect in a given clinical circumstance. In our review of pediatric psychopharmacology we are mainly concerned with the oral route. Once ingested the drug is absorbed from the gastrointestinal tract. The extent of drug absorption is influenced by the surface area available for drug absorption, and local blood flow. In addition the absorption also depends on the characteristics of the drug itself such as its water solubility, dosage form, or concentration.

Orally ingested drugs will undergo the first-pass effect before reaching the circulation (see below). The extent to which a drug is available at its site of action is referred to as the *bioavailability* of the drug.

Controlled-release preparations have been available for several psychotropic drugs, especially the stimulants. The basis for such a preparation is to control the rate of dissolution of the solid form of the drug in the gastrointestinal tract. The advantages of such preparations include a steady therapeutic level of the drug due to the elimination of peaks and troughs in drug concentrations and reduced frequency of administration (typically once daily). The interindividual variability of serum concentrations achieved is greater with controlled release preparations compared with immediate release forms; also failure of the dosage form may result in the release of the entire dose with consequent undesirable effects (dose dumping). Generally, controlled release forms are more appropriate for drugs with short half lives. Another route that is developed for some psychopharmacologic agents is the transdermal route using a patch (e.g. nicotine, methylphenidate, clonidine). The skin acts as a lipid membrane and drug absorption depends on the surface area exposed to drug, duration of exposure, and lipid solubility.

In order for the drug to exert its effect it has to reach the specific site of action and in order to do that the drug first needs to get across various cell membranes. The molecular size and shape of the drug, degree of ionization, solubility at site of absorption, and protein binding are some of the factors that influence the drug's ability to cross cellular membranes and reach the target sites of action. In *passive transport* across a cell membrane, the drug simply diffuses along a concentration gradient because of its lipid solubility properties. In *active transport* across a cell membrane, the drug is transported by an energy dependent carrier (sodium-potassium ATPase mechanism) against an electrochemical gradient. In the case of *facilitated diffusion* the drug is transported across the membrane by a nonenergy dependent carrier and in the direction of the concentration gradient.

Drug absorption from the intestine is influenced by drug characteristics such as its polarity and lipid solubility, degree of ionization, pKa of the drug, intestinal motility and transit time, and presence of other agents or food. Gastric effects including rate of dissolution, gastric pH and enzyme activity will also affect drug absorption. Crushing of the solid form and mixing it with food or liquids to make it more appropriate and palatable for children may also influence the absorption. Variation in transit time is of particular relevance for sustained release preparations.

## Distribution

Once absorbed, the drug reaches the bloodstream and is distributed to interstitial and intracellular fluids. In the blood many psychopharmacologic agents circulate bound to plasma protein (mainly albumin, alpha-1-glycoprotein, and lipoproteins). The extent of plasma protein binding is influenced by the concentration of drug in the blood, its affinity to the binding sites, and number of available binding sites. Extensive protein binding has the potential to lead to decreased metabolism and elimination of the drug. Such plasma protein binding is nonselective and another agent can potentially compete for the same binding sites and displace each other, changing the concentration of the unbound drug in the blood. The unbound drug is the only one available for its action. A change in the concentration of the unbound drug could lead to an increase or decrease in the effect of that drug. Some drugs may also be stored in tissues, for example, the storage and accumulation of lipid soluble drugs in the adipose tissue.

Unlike the distribution of the drug in various interstitial and intracellular fluids, the distribution of a drug into the central nervous system (CNS) requires it to first cross the blood–brain barrier (BBB). In the CNS the capillary endothelial cells form continuous tight junctions and along with the pericapillary glial cells constitute the BBB. Thus, in order to reach the CNS the drug must traverse across the endothelial cells and perivascular cell membranes. Similarly at the choroid plexus, epithelial cells form tight junctions. Therefore lipid solubility or the lipophilic property of the drug is an important factor that facilitates its transport across the BBB.

The *apparent volume of distribution* of a drug is defined as that volume of body fluid required to contain the entire amount of the drug in the body at the same measured concentration in the blood or the plasma. In other words it correlates the total amount of drug in the body to its concentration in the blood or plasma. The volume of drug distribution thus is a measure of its amount present in the extravascular tissues.

Volume of distribution value can be useful in determining the loading dose or dose needed to achieve the desired serum concentration of the drug [Loading dose = desired serum concentration of the drug (mg/L) × volume of distribution (L/kg) × patient's weight (kg)]. The volume of distribution of a given drug can vary significantly between children, adolescents, and adults, and between genders, because of differences in body composition. Other factors that influence such variability include age-related differences in protein binding capacity, cellular membrane permeability, hemodynamic factors, and concurrent disease states.

## Metabolism

Metabolism of a drug or its *biotransformation* generally converts it into a more water-soluble polar compound easy to excrete by the kidneys. The drug is converted into its inactive or active metabolites. Although liver is the primary site for metabolism of drugs, biotransformation can also occur to a lesser extent at other sites including the skin, lungs, intestine, and kidneys. Once ingested some of the drug may be metabolized in the intestinal epithelium or the liver into its inactive metabolites, thereby reducing the amount of drug that reaches the circulation (*the first pass effect*). *Bioavailability* of the drug refers to the drug that is available at its site of action and the fraction of the administered dose that is actually absorbed without undergoing the first pass effect.

In the liver, various enzyme systems metabolize drugs by two major pathways. *Phase I biotransformation reactions* typically involve hydrolysis, oxidation, reduction, and hydroxylation by enzyme systems on the endoplasmic reticulum, whereas *phase II reactions* involve conjugation with glucuronic acid (or glutathione, sulfate, or acetate) by enzyme systems in the cytoplasm. The cytochrome P450 (CYP450) enzymes, which are involved in Phase I oxidative reactions, play an important role in the biotransformation of drugs with wide-ranging therapeutic and drug interaction implications. The genetic variability in CYP450 enzymes can account for clinically significant interindividual variability in drug effects. Other factors affecting biotransformation include concurrent disease states, age, and the presence of other drugs. These factors have the potential to increase the effect of a drug, decrease its efficacy, or increase its toxicity. Specific updated sources (http://www.medicine.iupui.edu/flockhart/; http://www.genetest.com/human_p450_database/index.html.p450+; www.mhc.com/Cytochrome/) should be consulted to check for the possibility of such effects and drug-drug interactions related to CYP450 system. Manufacturer's product information should also be reviewed to check for drug-drug interactions (http://www.epocrates.com/; http://www.pdr.net).

When there is saturation of the protein binding sites, the capacity of the liver to further metabolize the drug or the capacity of the kidneys to excrete the drug follows the principles of *nonlinear pharmacokinetics*.

Overall children metabolize drugs that use hepatic pathways more efficiently and therefore need a higher dose and more frequent daily dosing.

## Excretion

Polar (hydrophilic) compounds are excreted more efficiently by the kidneys. Some drugs may be excreted unchanged whereas others, particularly the lipid-soluble drugs, are first metabolized to more polar water-soluble compounds before being excreted by the kidneys. Renal excretion may vary depending upon the age of the patient and the efficiency of the renal function. Children have more efficient renal elimination of drugs compared with adults.

*Clearance* of a drug is a measure of the body's efficiency in eliminating the drug. A *steady state concentration of drug* is reached when the rate of drug elimination equals the rate of drug administration. Thus the dosing rate is the product of clearance and steady state concentration of the drug. The rate of clearance of a given drug remains constant over a range of its measured blood (body fluid) concentrations. When a constant fraction of drug in the body is eliminated per unit of time it is said to follow *first-order kinetics*. In first-order kinetics the elimination rate is proportional to the concentration of the drug in the plasma. When the metabolic system for drug elimination is saturated, a fixed amount of drug is eliminated per unit of time and it is said to follow *zero-order kinetics*. In zero-order kinetics, clearance will vary with the drug concentration.

The *half-life* of a drug is defined as the time it takes for the plasma concentration (or the amount of drug in the body) to be reduced by 50% and it varies depending upon the clearance and volume of distribution of the drug. Generally, half-life is a clinically useful indicator of the time required for the drug to reach steady state ($\sim$ four half-lives), the time that will be required to eliminate the drug from the body, and a mechanism by which to estimate the dosing interval.

## Drug dosing and therapeutic drug monitoring

The knowledge of the pharmacokinetic parameters of a drug is applied clinically in determining the appropriate dose and dose interval for the drug to achieve desired concentration and realize its therapeutic effect. For many drugs a relationship exists between the measured level of the drug in the body fluid and its therapeutic effects; whereas for many others such a relationship is not clear. Some of the pharmacokinetic concepts useful in designing the optimum dosing regimen and therapeutic drug monitoring include clearance, apparent volume of distribution, elimination half-life, and bioavailability of the drug, reviewed above.

A drug's concentration in the body that is within a range that provides optimal efficacy without undue side effects or toxicity defines the *therapeutic window* for that drug. The strategy for dosage determination of a drug based on the relationship between its serum or plasma concentration and desired therapeutic effects (or toxic effects) is referred to as the *target concentration strategy*.

In order to *maintain* a desired therapeutic level or the steady state concentration, the drug should be administered at a rate that equals its rate of elimination. A drug dose and dosing interval can be calculated based on the desired concentration of the drug, its clearance, and bioavailability. A *loading* dose is typically reserved for cases where a rapid action of the drug is desired. A large loading dose may be associated with undesirable toxicity in some patients, and for drugs with long half lives it will take a long time for the drug to clear from the body.

It is important to understand that most recommended dosage ranges are designed for an average patient with a given disorder and there is considerable interindividual (genetic) variability in pharmacokinetics and pharmacodynamics; pharmacokinetics is also affected by any associated disease states. Because of lack of sufficient clinical trials and data, the drug dosage of many agents used in children and adolescents are extrapolated based on studies in adult subjects. Therefore individualization of the dosage is the most prudent approach, starting with a low dose and gradually titrating up to achieve the desired effects.

Not all drugs have a clear correlation between their measured concentration in blood (or body fluid) and the desired therapeutic effects; however in many instances therapeutic drug monitoring can be useful to guide the treatment. The drug concentration just prior to the next dose is due (i.e. the trough level) is the most useful to guide any adjustment of the dose during the initiation as well as the maintenance phase of therapy. When the same dose of the drug is given at the same dosage intervals, a steady state is reached after four half-lives. In cases where no loading dose is given and a drug has a narrow therapeutic window with concern for toxicity, the initial drug concentration should be measured after at least 2 half-lives in order to assess the need to adjust the dose. Another level should then be measured after 2 more half-lives (that is after a total of four half-lives). A pharmacokinetic consultation is valuable where available for appropriate individualization of the dosage regimen. Given the difficulties with therapeutic monitoring of drugs it is neither necessary nor useful in all cases; rather individualization based on regular clinical assessment is more useful and desirable in most cases.

# ■ Pharmacodynamics

*Pharmacodynamics* in simple terms refers to the effects of the drug on the body and in broad terms encompasses the concepts of sites of drug action, the structure activity relationship, various types of receptors, the drug-receptor interactions, concepts of specificity and selectivity of drug action, and mechanisms of drug action. In our discussion of the psychopharmacological agents these and other related concepts are reviewed in the context of chemical neurotransmission below.

# ■ Neurotransmission

## The neuron

The main components of a neuron or nerve cell are the cell body or soma, an axon, and the dendrites (Figure 2.1). Each neuron is enclosed in a neuronal membrane. The nucleus, the rough endoplasmic reticulum, the smooth endoplasmic reticulum, the Golgi apparatus, and the mitochondria are contained within the cell body (Figure 2.2). The ribosomes on the rough endoplasmic reticulum and the free ribosomes are the major sites for protein synthesis directed by the messenger ribonucleic acid (mRNA). The function of smooth endoplasmic reticulum varies depending upon its location and includes its role in finessing the protein structure and regulating concentration of certain intracellular chemicals. The Golgi apparatus plays a major role in chemical processing of the proteins. The mitochondrion is the site of cellular respiration and provides the chemical energy for the intracellular biochemical reactions. The neuronal cell membrane is a dynamic complex structure that wraps over the cytoskeleton of

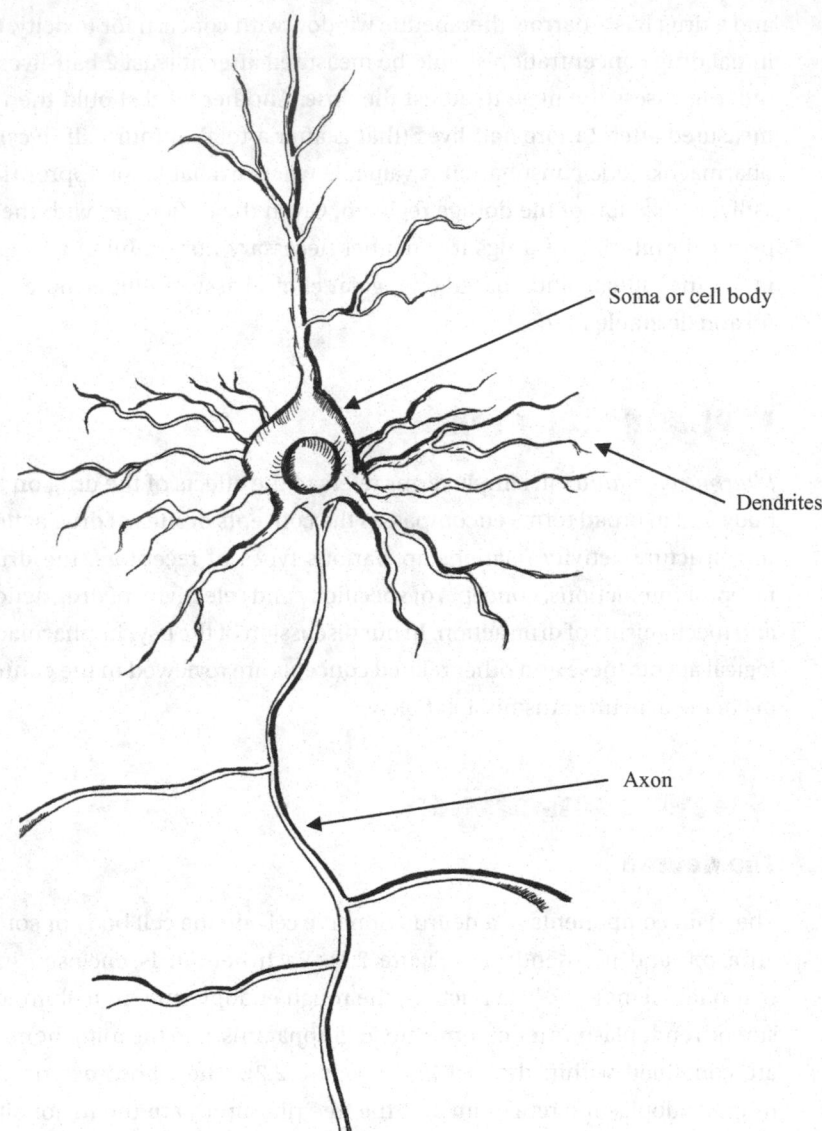

Soma or cell body

Dendrites

Axon

**Figure 2.1** Basic structure of a neuron.

the cell consisting of microtubules, microfilaments, and neurofilaments. Specific genes are located on the deoxyribonucleic acid (DNA) in each chromosome inside the nucleus.

In addition to the structures of the cell body, the neuron is uniquely characterized by the axonal and dendritic processes. Each axon has three main

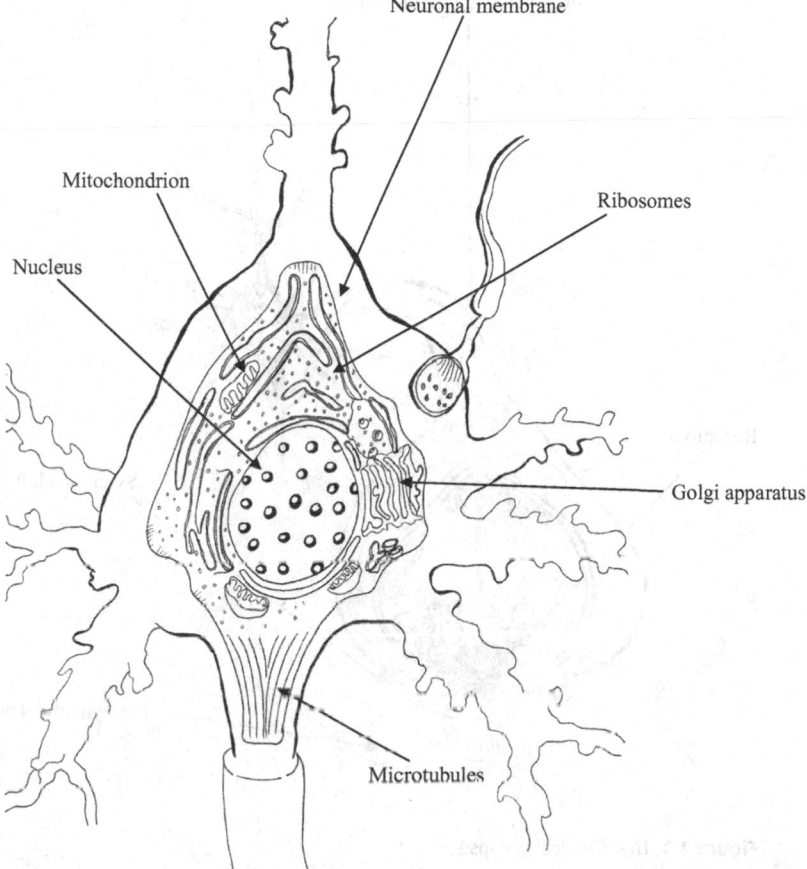

Neuronal membrane

Mitochondrion

Ribosomes

Nucleus

Golgi apparatus

Microtubules

**Figure 2.2** Basic internal structure of a neuron.

parts, the axon hillock, the axon proper, and the axon terminal. The point of contact between the presynaptic axon terminal and the postsynaptic dentrite is called the *synapse*. Axon terminal may also end on the cell body of the postsynaptic neuron. Neurotransmitter is stored in the synaptic vesicles in the axon terminal. Axons carry the neuronal impulse to various other neurons in the brain. The information or input is carried to the cell body of the receiving neuron. On the receiving end the information or impulse is received at the dendrites.

## The synapse

At the synapse (Figure 2.3) the electrical impulse from the presynaptic neuron is converted to a chemical signal that is carried to the postsynaptic

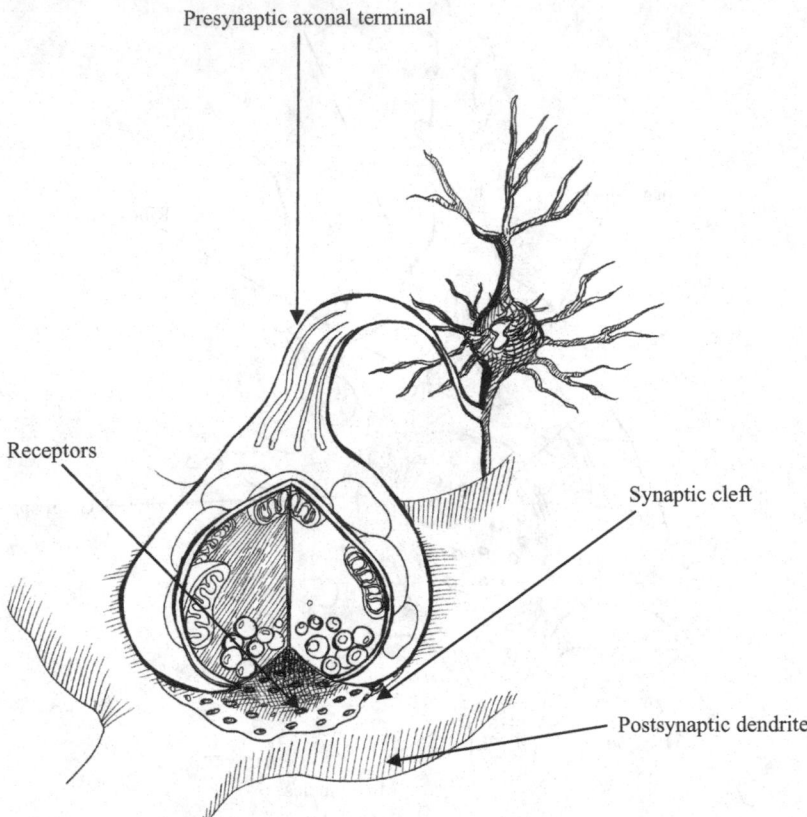

Presynaptic axonal terminal

Receptors

Synaptic cleft

Postsynaptic dendrite

**Figure 2.3** The chemical synapse.

receptors where it is again converted to an electrical impulse in the postsynaptic neuron.

There are two types of neuronal synapses: electrical and chemical. The electrical synapses are located at gap junctions and allow free bidirectional movement of ions across cell membranes. Their function in the brain varies at different sites; they provide for fast transmission of impulses. Most of the synaptic transmission in the brain occurs at the chemical synapses. Autoreceptors are membrane-bound receptors on the presynaptic membrane and regulate the release and in some cases synthesis of the intrinsic neurotransmitter. Certain other receptors on the presynaptic membrane can be modulated by neurotransmitters from nearby neurons and are called heteroreceptors.

The membrane-bound postsynaptic neuroreceptors can generally be classified into two types: (1) Transmitter-gated (or ligand-gated) ion

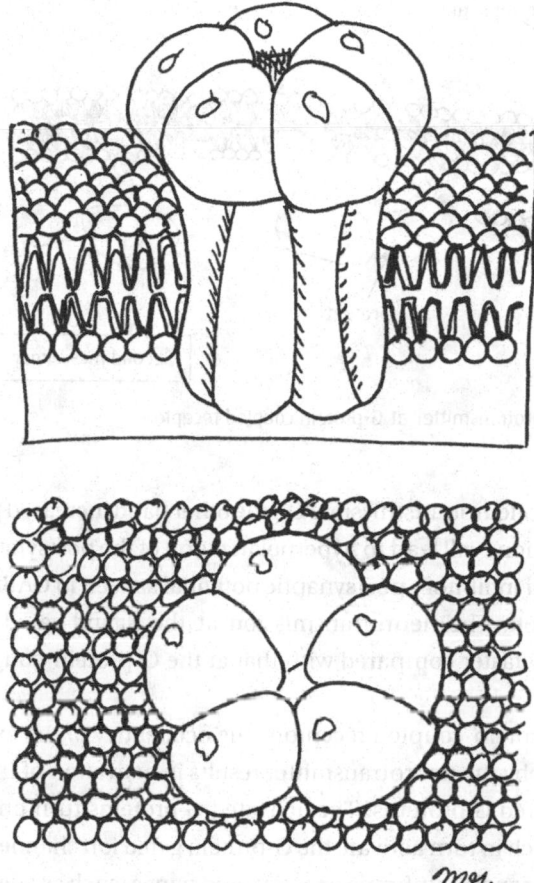

**Figure 2.4** Structure of a transmitter-gated ion channel as it appears from a side view (upper figure) and from the top (lower figure) showing the central pore surrounded by five subunits.

channels (Figure 2.4), and (2) G-protein-coupled receptors (Figure 2.5). A transmitter- or ligand-gated ion channel receptor consists of five subunits that are arranged as columns in a circle thus forming a pore or a channel in the middle. The neurotransmitter binds to the specific site on the extracelluar portion of the receptor, leading to opening of the channel. The effect on the postsynaptic neuron depends on which ion is preferentially passed through the channel into the postsynaptic neuron. Movement of *sodium* ions into the postsynaptic neuron results in depolarization of the postsynaptic cell and generation of excitatory postsynaptic potential as

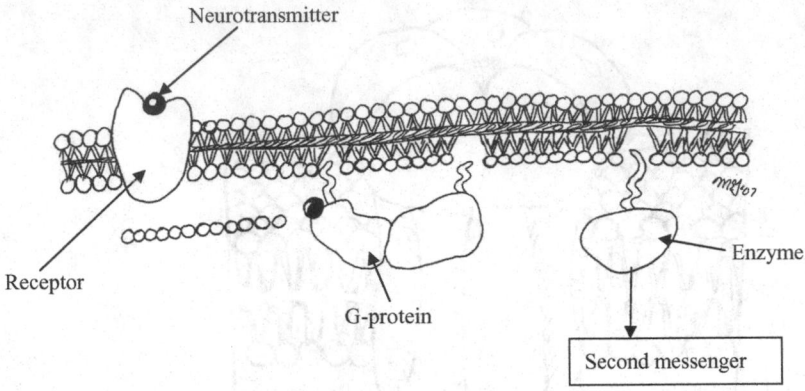

**Figure 2.5** Action of neurotransmitter at G-protein coupled receptors.

seen in glutamatergic neurotransmission. On the other hand increased permeability to *chloride* ions will lead to hyperpolarization of the postsynaptic cell and generation of inhibitory postsynaptic potential as seen in GABAergic neurotransmission. The neurotransmission at the ligand-gated ion channels is relatively faster compared with that at the G-protein-coupled receptors.

In the case of G-protein-coupled receptors, the occupancy of the extracellular receptor site by the neurotransmitter results in activation of intracellular receptor-linked G proteins. The activated G proteins turn on the effector proteins which in turn activate the G-protein gated ion channels in the postsynaptic neuronal membrane or activate enzymes (such as adenylyl cyclase and phospholipase C) to form intracellular second messengers. Second messengers then lead to a biochemical cascade eventually communicating the message to the DNA of the postsynaptic neuron. Because of their metabolic effects, the G-protein-coupled receptors are also known as metabotropic receptors.

## Chemical neurotransmission

Chemical neurotransmission is mediated by specific neurotransmitters in the brain, and a large number of these have been identified. There are various classes of neurotransmitters in the CNS; amine and monoamines are of interest in our review of psychopharmacology. Other classes of neurotransmitters, not reviewed here, use different pathways for synthesis, storage, release, and ways of communication. Still others follow non-synaptic neu-rotransmission.

Synthesis of different neurotransmitters in the presynaptic neuron varies to some extent for specific neurotransmitters utilizing specific amino acids and enzymes. Neurotransmitter synthesis is directed by mRNA and occurs in the cytosol of the axon terminal (Figure 2.6). The amine and amino acid neurotransmitters are then taken into synaptic vesicles by specialized trans-porter proteins. The neurotransmitter is stored in the synaptic vesicles in the axonal terminal until it is released into the synaptic cleft.

The peptide neurotransmitters are assembled from the amino acids in the rough endoplasmic reticulum and the active neurotransmitter segment is split in the Golgi apparatus. The secretory granules containing the active peptide then are carried to the axon terminal.

A nerve impulse or action potential in the axon terminal triggers the release of a specific neurotransmitter into the synaptic cleft. Depolariza-tion of the cell membrane results in activation of the voltage-gated cal-cium channels – the active zones open, allowing influx of calcium ions into the presynaptic axon terminal. The synaptic vesicle is anchored to the cell membrane and the neurotransmitter is spilled into the synaptic cleft, a pro-cess called exocytosis (Figure 2.7). The process of recovery of the synaptic vesicle membrane after the neurotransmitter is released from the vesicle is called endocytosis. Once released into the synaptic cleft, the neurotrans-mitters can be either destroyed by enzymes or transported back into the presynaptic axon terminal by membrane-bound neurotransmitter specific transporters.

Postsynaptic receptor occupancy by the neurotransmitter initiates the postsynaptic neurotransmission process. It is thus understood that the elec-trical nerve impulse in the presynaptic neuron is converted by excitation-secretion coupling into a chemical signal.

Postsynaptic receptor occupancy by the neurotransmitter (first messen-ger) results in the activation or formation of the second messenger in the postsynaptic neuron. Cyclic adenosine monophosphate (cAMP) and phosphatidyl inositol are examples of second messengers. The second messenger triggers a biochemical cascade and synthesis of various ele-ments including the transcription factors.

Each gene typically has a coding region and a regulatory region. The regulatory region has an enhancer element and a promoter element. The coding region on the DNA has the template for the corresponding RNA.

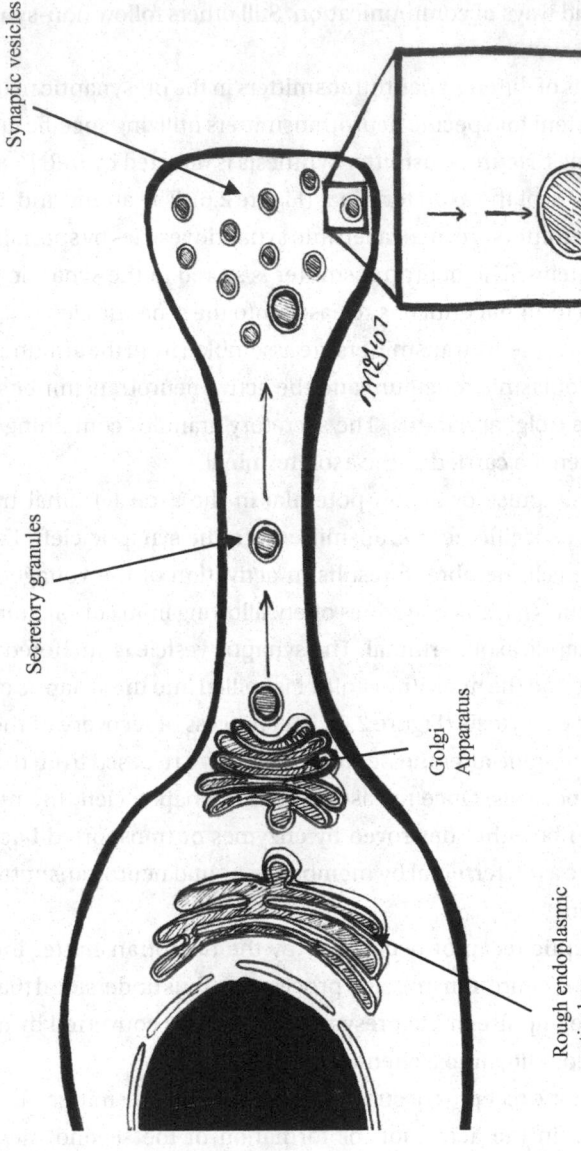

**Figure 2.6** The synthesis and release of neurotransmitters.

Synaptic vesicles

Secretory granules

Golgi
Apparatus

Rough endoplasmic
reticulum

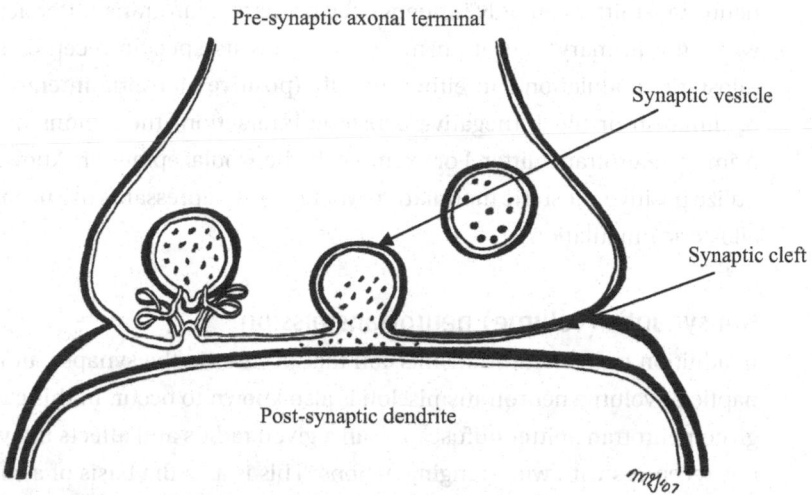

**Figure 2.7** Release of neurotransmitter by exocytosis.

Transcription factors activated by phosphorylation bind to the promoter region of the DNA, in turn activating the enzyme RNA polymerase. The action of activated RNA polymerase on the coding region results in the formation of messenger RNA (mRNA). The process of mRNA formation from DNA template is called transcription and the mRNA is called the transcript. Certain noncoding regions (introns) on the DNA transcribed onto the initial mRNA are removed by the process of RNA splicing leaving only the coding sequences (exons) in the mRNA. Messenger RNA leaves the nucleus and reaches various sites in the neuron to initiate protein synthesis. The process of assembling various amino acids to create specific proteins as directed by the mRNA is called translation.

These proteins are the building blocks for various elements in the post-synaptic neuron with specialized functions, including neurotransmitter receptors, the ion channels, various peptides and enzymes, transcription factors, neurotransmitter transporter, and neurotropic growth factors. The regulation of gene expression also affects the process of synaptogenesis.

## Allosteric modulation

When a neurotransmitter (primary) occupies its specific receptor site, it triggers the postsynaptic chemical neurotransmission. When a different neurotransmitter (secondary) occupies its receptor site and indirectly influences the primary neuroreceptor transmission it is said to be modulating the primary neurotransmitter action allosterically. The secondary neurotransmitter can only influence the primary neurotransmitter action when the primary neurotransmitter occupies its specific receptor site. Allosteric modulation can either amplify (positive allosteric interaction) or diminish or block (negative allosteric interaction) the actions of the primary neurotransmitter. For example the benzodiazepines are known to utilize positive allosteric modulation whereas antidepressants use negative allosteric modulation.

## Nonsynaptic (volume) neurotransmission

In addition to the neurotransmission that occurs via the synapse, nonsynaptic or volume neurotransmission is also known to occur. In this case a given neurotransmitter diffuses within a given radius and affects the various receptors with wide-ranging actions. This is also the basis of a single drug acting on different receptors with different actions.

## Divergence and convergence

A given neurotransmitter can activate multiple subtypes of receptors each mediating a different function. In fact, this ability of a neurotransmitter, referred to as divergence, is a common phenomenon, exemplified by glutamate. On the other hand different neurotransmitters acting on their specific receptors can activate a particular effector system, a phenomenon called convergence. Neurons also have the ability to integrate both the divergent and convergent systems.

## Agonists and antagonists

Naturally occurring neurotransmitters stimulate the receptors on which they bind and are thus said to be agonists. Similarly pharmacological agents that stimulate specific receptors are also called *agonists*. Antagonist agents block the actions of agonists. Antagonists do not have any intrinsic activity of their own but in the presence of an agonist they block its activity. *Antagonists* also will block the actions of inverse agonist and partial agonist as well. A pharmacologic agent that binds to a receptor resulting in action that is opposite of agonist is called an *inverse agonist*. The action of an inverse agonist is not dependent on the presence of an agonist. *Partial agonist* binding to a specific receptor will have action that is similar but relatively weaker to that of an agonist.

# ■ Major neurotransmitter systems

## Cholinergic system

Acetylcholine (ACh) is the neurotransmitter used in the cholinergic system. Acetylcholine is synthesized in the cholinergic neurons by the interaction of choline and acetyl coenzyme A mediated by the enzyme choline acetyltransferase. Acetylcholine is stored in the vesicles in the presynaptic neuron until it is released by appropriate nerve impulse into the synaptic cleft. From the synaptic cleft acetylcholine can either be transported back into the presynaptic neuron by the acetylcholine transporter or destroyed by the enzyme acetyl cholinesterase (AChE). Because the acetylcholine is destroyed by the acetyl cholinesterase rapidly, it is mainly the choline that is transported back into the neuron and reused to synthesize acetylcholine again.

Another enzyme called pseudocholinesterase or butyrylcholinesterase can also inactivate ACh especially in the glial cells. In addition to the cholinergic neurons, ACh is also present in various other sites in the body including skeletal muscle and blood cells.

Various types of muscarinic and nicotinic receptors are the major sub-types of cholinergic receptors; muscarinic receptors are G-protein linked whereas nicotinic receptors are ligand-gated ion channels.

The cell bodies of the cholinergic neurons are located between the septum and the nucleus basalis of Meynert in the basal forebrain with projections to the hippocampus, amygdala, and cortex. These pathways are believed to mediate memory, learning, problem-solving abilities, novelty seeking, sleep–wake cycles, and judgement. Drugs that inhibit AChE prevent the destruction of ACh and subsequently increase ACh concentration.

## Dopaminergic system

The monoamine dopamine is the neurotransmitter of the dopaminergic system. Dopamine is synthesized from its precursor amino acid tyrosine which is converted to dihydrophenylalanine (DOPA) by tyrosine hydroxylase. DOPA is converted to dopamine by DOPA decarboxylase. Once synthesized in the presynaptic nerve terminal, dopamine is packaged in the vesicles for storage. Presynaptic action potential triggers the release of dopamine from the vesicles into the synaptic cleft. Dopamine can be metabolized by the enzymes monoamine oxidase (MAO) or catechol-ortho-methyl-transaminase (COMT). Dopamine is also transported back from the synaptic cleft into the presynaptic terminal by presynaptic dopamine specific transporters, where it can be repackaged into vesicles and stored for future use. Dopamine transporter is a target for drug action (e.g. stimulants).

Five subtypes of dopamine receptors have been described namely D1–D5, present both on the presynaptic neuron as well as on the postsynaptic neuron. Presynaptic receptors act as autoreceptors whereas dopamine occupation of the postsynaptic receptors activates second messenger system and postsynaptic events. Different subtypes of dopamine receptors predominantly express themselves in specific regions or sites in the brain, thereby influencing specific functions. Postsynaptic receptors are targets for dopamine antagonist drugs (e.g. antipsychotic agents).

Dopamine pathways from substantia nigra projecting to caudate and putamen modulate GABAergic neurons and their imbalance leads to extrapyramidal symptoms (such as tremors). Those from the ventral tegmental area projecting to the mesolimbic system (amygdala, nucleus accumbens) are implicated in the development of addiction. The pathways from the ventral tegmental area to mesocortical system are involved in "fine tuning" of cortical neurons and their function is improved by stimulants. The projections from hypothalamus to pituitary play a role in prolactin release and neuroleptic blockade leads to hyperprolactinemia. The effects of dopamine blockade are listed in Table 7.3 (see Chapter 7).

## The GABAergic system

The amino acid gamma-amino butyric acid (GABA) is the neurotransmitter used in GABAergic neurotransmission. GABA is synthesized in the GABAergic neurons from its precursor glutamate by action of the enzyme glutamate decarboxylase. GABA is stored in the presynaptic vesicles until released into the synaptic cleft following appropriate nerve impulse. The released GABA can be either destroyed by GABA transaminase or transported back into the presynaptic terminal by GABA-specific presynaptic transporter for repackaging and storage for reuse. GABA is the main inhibitory neurotransmitter in the CNS.

Two GABA receptor subtypes have been identified, namely GABA-A and GABA-B. The role of GABA-B receptor is limited to its binding specifically with the muscle relaxant baclofen. Postsynaptic GABA-A receptors belong to the superfamily of ligand-gated ion channel receptors. Receptor occupancy by GABA opens the ion channel and allows increased conductance of chloride ions into the neuron leading to fast neurotransmission and inhibitory action. The GABAergic system exerts inhibitory control over the glutamatergic system and the balance between the two systems allows for normal neuronal function.

GABAergic neurons are widespread in the CNS and spinal cord, with interneurons in the cortex, and medium- to long-range projections, including: caudate nucleus and putamen to globus pallidus; globus pallidus to thalamus and substantia nigra; septum to hippocampus; and substantia nigra to superior colliculus.

Benzodiazepine receptors are located at sites nearby the GABA-A receptors. Different subtypes of benzodiazepine receptors are predominantly found at various locations in the CNS and thought to mediate specific functions. Benzodiazepine receptors allosterically modulate the GABA-A receptors. In addition to benzodiazepine receptors various other receptors are located nearby GABA-A receptors. Thus, the interaction of these various receptors is involved in mediating the effects of benzodiazepine agents.

## Glutamatergic system

Glutamate is the predominant excitatory neurotransmitter in the CNS. Glutamate is synthesized in the neuron by conversion of glutamine to glutamate by the enzyme glutaminase. Glutamate is stored in the presynaptic vesicles until it is released into the synaptic cleft. Glial cells near the neuron also supply glutamine to the neuron for glutamate synthesis. Once glutamate is released into the synaptic cleft it binds to the postsynaptic receptors initiating postsynaptic excitation. Glutamate is removed from the synaptic cleft by the presynaptic transporter back into the synaptic terminal, as well as by a glial transporter into the nearby glial cell.

The major glutamate receptor subtypes include N-methyl-d-aspartate (NMDA), alpha-amino-3-hydroxy-5-methyl-isoxazole-4-propionic acid (AMPA), and kainate, which are linked to ion channel; and a metabotropic glutamate receptor subtype that is G-protein linked involved in long-term potentiation and memory formation.

One of the receptors believed to mediate the excitotoxicity associated with glutamatergic neurotransmission is the NMDA receptor. Several other nearby receptors are believed to be involved in allosteric modulation of the

NMDA receptor complex. Stimulation of the NMDA receptor site allows increased conductance of calcium ions into the neuron and trigger postsynaptic excitatory neurotransmission. Glutamatergic excitation represents the spectrum from normal excitation to too much excitation resulting in neuronal damage. Glutamatergic excitotoxicity is believed to play a major role in the pathophysiology of neurodegenerative diseases, seizures, and stroke. Decreased glutamate on the other hand can lead to psychosis.

NMDA receptors in the hippocampus are associated with long-term memory. Glutamatergic neurons are widely distributed in the CNS and include various interconnection pathways in the cerebral cortex, the extra pyramidal system, the pyramidal system, and thalamocortical system.

## Noradrenergic system

Monoamine norepinephrine is the neurotransmitter for noradrenergic neurons. Norepinephrine (NE) is synthesized from its precursor amino acid tyrosine in the cell body or axonal nerve terminal. Tyrosine is converted to dihydrophenylalanine (DOPA) by tyrosine hydroxylase. DOPA is then converted to dopamine by DOPA decarboxylase. Dopamine is converted to norepinephrine by dopamine beta-hydroxylase.

Once synthesized, the NE is packaged into vesicles where it is stored until released into the synaptic cleft during noradrenergic transmission. From the synaptic cleft the NE can be transported back into the presynaptic nerve terminal by NE specific transporters. Norepinephrine thus recovered is repackaged into storage vesicles for future use. Norepinephrine is also destroyed by the enzymes monoamine oxidase (MAO) predominantly located in the mitochondria; and catechol-ortho-methyl-transaminase (COMT) predominantly located in the postsynaptic neuron.

Once NE is released from the presynaptic neuron into the synaptic cleft, it occupies the NE-specific postsynaptic receptors. Norepinephrine receptors are classified into alpha-1, alpha-2, beta-1, and beta-2 subtypes. Alpha-2 receptor subtype is present on the presynaptic axon terminal (terminal alpha-2 receptor) and in the cell body and nearby dendrites (somatodendritic alpha-2 receptor). The presynaptic alpha-2 receptors regulate the release of NE and thus act as autoreceptors. Alpha-1, alpha-2, beta-1, and beta-2 receptors are present on the postsynaptic membrane. Postsynaptic receptor occupation by NE triggers postsynaptic events including second messenger activation and gene expression.

The cell bodies for noradrenergic neurons are predominantly located in the locus coeruleus in the brainstem. Different noradrenergic projections from locus coeruleus are involved in specific effects of NE including regulation of mood, attention, vigilance, cognition, emotions, information processing, working memory, energy, and movements. Norepinephrine deficiency syndrome is characterized by impaired attention, difficulty in concentrating, impaired working memory, decreased speed of information processing, depressed mood, fatigue, and psychomotor retardation. Different functions are regulated by a different subtype of NE receptor in the CNS.

Actions of NE outside of the CNS mediated via different pathways include regulation of blood pressure, heart rate, and bladder emptying.

## Serotonergic system

Serotonin or 5-hydroxytryptamine (5-HT) is synthesized in the presynaptic axon terminal from its precursor tryptophan. Tryptophan is first converted to 5-hydroxytryptophan by the action of tryptophan hydroxylase. 5-hydroxytryptophan is then converted to 5-hydroxytryptamine by the action of aromatic amino acid decarboxylase.

Serotonin is stored in the presynaptic vesicle until released by the presynaptic terminal into the synaptic cleft. Serotonin can be destroyed by monoamine oxidase and also transported back into the presynaptic terminal by serotonin transporters. There are several 5-HT receptor subtypes. Presynaptic receptors act as autoreceptors. In addition to 5-HT autoreceptors, the presynaptic serotonergic terminal also has alpha-2 noradrenergic heteroreceptors responsive to NE. Thus serotonin release can be blocked in part by NE via its action on the alpha-2 noradrenergic heteroreceptors. On the other hand the action of NE on the alpha-1 adrenergic heteroreceptors present on the presynaptic cell body triggers release of serotonin. Thus there is both an inhibitory and excitatory interaction between the noradrenergic and serotonergic systems.

The cell bodies of serotonergic neurons are located in the raphe nucleus in the brain stem. Various projections to different areas in the brain, brain stem, and spinal cord from raphe nucleus (including amygdala and hippocampus) are associated with various specific 5-HT receptor subtypes and specific functions attributed to serotonin. Deficiency of serotonin is clinically characterized by depressed mood, anxiety, panic attacks, phobias, obsessions, compulsions, and food craving.

# ■ Summary

Important developmental differences exist between children and adults in terms of drug pharmacokinetics and pharmacodynamics that have significant implications for dosing, therapeutic effects, and toxicity. It is generally prudent to start at a low dosage and gradually titrate higher; however the dosages required for therapeutic effects in children often are similar to those used in adults. Use of multiple drugs should generally be avoided but the presence of comorbid disorders is quite common necessitating the use of a combination of drugs. It is recognized that the immature or still maturing brain is more sensitive to the effects of a given drug and long-term implications are not clearly elucidated; at the same time the hepatic metabolism and renal excretion are relatively more efficient in children that eliminate the drug. The side effects between children and adults also vary; children tend to experience relatively more behavioral and cognitive side effects whereas adults tend to experience more somatic side effects.

Receptors, enzymes, and processes of neurotransmission are targets of drug action as well as causes of mental and neurological disorders. The various elements of the neurotransmission systems can be modulated not only by pharmacological agents but also are constantly changing because of the ongoing neuromaturation and experience (including psychotherapy) throughout childhood and adolescence. Neuroplasticity of the synaptic system is an important consideration in the pathophysiology and recovery or treatment of mental and neurological disorders in children and adolescents. Pharmacological agents can have acute as well as long-term effects on the processes of neurotransmission. Some of the therapeutic effects as well as side effects can be explained by acute changes in the levels of neurotransmitter or the long-term alterations in responses of the postsynaptic neuron.

## SELECTED BIBLIOGRAPHY

Allison C, Pratt JA. 2003. Neuroadaptive processes in GABAergic and glutamatergic systems in benzodiazepine dependence. *Pharmacol. Ther.*, 98(2):171–95.

Bear MF, Connors BW, Paradiso MA. 2007. *Neuroscience: Exploring the Brain, 3rd edn.* Baltimore: Lippincott Williams & Wilkins.

Beleboni RO, Carolino RO, Pizzo AB *et al.* 2004. Pharmacological and biochemical aspects of GABAergic neurotransmission: pathological and neuropsychobiological relationships. *Cell Mol. Neurobiol.*, 24(6):707–28.

Berridge CW, Waterhouse BD. 2003. The locus coeruleus-noradrenergic system: modulation of behavioral state and state-dependent cognitive processes. *Brain Res. Brain Res. Rev.*, 42(1):33–84.

Braithwaite SP, Paul S, Nairn AC, Lombroso PJ. 2006. Synaptic plasticity: one STEP at a time. *Trends Neurosci.*, 29(8):452–8.

Brambilla P, Perez J, Barale F, Schettini G, Soares JC. 2003. GABAergic dysfunction in mood disorders. *Mol. Psychiatry*, 8(8):721–37.

Buxton ILO. 2006. Pharmacokinetics and pharmacodynamics: The dynamics of drug absorption, distribution, action, and elimination. In Brunton L, Parker K, Lazo J, Buxton I, Blumenthal D (Eds.) *Goodman & Gilman's The Pharmacological Basis of Therapeutics, 11th edn.* New York: McGraw Hill Medical.

Celine F, Ouissame MF, Nasser H. 2006. Long-term adaptive changes induced by serotonergic antidepressant drugs. *Expert Rev. Neurother.*, 6(2):235–45.

Centonze D, Gubellini P, Pisani A, Bernardi G, Calabresi P. 2003. Dopamine, acetyl-choline and nitric oxide systems interact to induce corticostriatal synaptic plasticity. *Rev. Neurosci.*, 14(3):207–16.

Chen HS, Lipton SA. 2006. The chemical biology of clinically tolerated NMDA receptor antagonists. *J. Neurochem.*, 97(6):1611–26.

Cooke SF, Bliss TV. 2006. Plasticity in the human central nervous system. *Brain*, 129 (Pt 7):1659–73.

Damsa C, Bumb A, Bianchi-Demicheli F *et al.* 2004. "Dopamine-dependent" side effects of selective serotonin reuptake inhibitors: a clinical review. *J. Clin. Psychiatry* 65(8):1064–8.

Dujardin K, Laurent B. 2003. Dysfunction of the human memory systems: role of the dopaminergic transmission. *Curr. Opin. Neurol.*, 16 (Suppl. 2):S11–6.

Ferraguti F, Shigemoto R. 2006. Metabotropic glutamate receptors. *Cell Tissue Res.*, 326(2):483–504.

Filip M, Frankowska M, Zaniewska M, Golda A, Przegalinski E. 2005. The serotonergic system and its role in cocaine addiction. *Pharmacol. Rep.*, 57(6):685–700.

Fritschy JM, Brunig I. 2003. Formation and plasticity of GABAergic synapses: physiological mechanisms and pathophysiological implications. *Pharmacol. Ther.*, 98(3):299–323.

Greene JG. 2006. Gene expression profiles of brain dopamine neurons and relevance to neuropsychiatric disease. *J. Physiol.*, 1; 575(Part 2):411–16.

Greenhill LL, Tosyali MC. 1998. Child and adolescent psychopharmacology: Important developmental issues. *Pediatr. Clin. N. Am.*, 45(5):1021–36.

Hensler JG. 2006. Serotonergic modulation of the limbic system. *Neurosci. Biobehav. Rev.*, 30(2):203–14.

Heresco-Levy U. 2005. Glutamatergic neurotransmission modulators as emerging new drugs for schizophrenia. *Expert Opin Emerg. Drugs*, 10(4):827–44.

Johnston, GA. 2005. GABA(A) receptor channel pharmacology. *Curr. Pharm. Des.*, 11(15):1867–85.

Kienast T, Heinz A. 2006. Dopamine and the diseased brain. *CNS Neurol Disord Drug Targets*, 5(1):109–31.

Lee FJ, Wang YT, Liu F. 2005. Direct receptor cross-talk can mediate the modulation of excitatory and inhibitory neurotransmission by dopamine. *J. Mol. Neurosci.*, 26(2–3):245–52.

Lujan R, Shigemoto R, Lopez-Bendito G. 2005. Glutamate and GABA receptor signaling in the developing brain. *Neuroscience*, 130(3):567–80.

Majewska AK, Sur M. 2006. Plasticity and specificity of cortical processing networks. *Trends Neurosci.*, 29(6):323–9.

Mangina CA, Sokolov EN. 2006. Neuronal plasticity in memory and learning abilities: theoretical position and selective review. *Int. J. Psychophysiol.*, 60(3):203–14.

Marien MR, Colpaert FC, Rosenquist AC. 2004. Noradrenergic mechanisms in neurodegenerative diseases: a theory. *Brain Res. Brain Res. Rev.*, 45(1):38–78.

Meredith CW, Jaffe C, Ang-Lee K, Saxon AJ. 2005. Implications of chronic methamphetamine use: a literature review. *Harv. Rev. Psychiatry*, 13(3):141–54.

Middlemiss DN, Price GW, Watson JM. 2002. Serotonergic targets in depression. *Curr. Opin. Pharmacol.*, 2(1):18–22.

Mody I, Pearce RA. 2004. Diversity of inhibitory neurotransmission through GABA(A) receptors. *Trends Neurosci.*, 27(9); 569–75.

Pallas SL, Wenner P, Gonzalez-Islas C. *et al.* 2006. Developmental plasticity of inhibitory circuitry. *J. Neurosci.*, 26(41):10358–61.

Pinheiro P, Mulle C. 2006. Kainate receptors. *Cell Tissue Res.*, 326(2):457–82.

Rollenhagen A, Lubke JH. 2006. The morphology of excitatory central synapses: from structure to function. *Cell Tissue Res.*, 326(2):221–37.

Sanger DJ. 2004. The search for novel antipsychotics: pharmacological and molecular targets. *Expert Opin. Ther. Targets*, 8(6):631–41.

Scheffer RF. 2006. Psychopharmacology: Clinical implications of brain neurochemistry. *Pediatr. Clin. N. Am.*, 53:767–75.

Schmitz Y, Benoit-Marand M, Gonon F, Sulzer D. 2003. Presynaptic regulation of dopaminergic neurotransmission. *J. Neurochem.*, 87(2):273–89.

Sem'yanov AV. 2005. Diffusional extrasynaptic neurotransmission via glutamate and GABA. *Neurosci. Behav. Physiol.*, 35(3):253–66.

Sprengel R. 2006. Role of AMPA receptors in synaptic plasticity. *Cell Tissue Res.*, 326(2):447–55.

Stahl DM. 2000. *Essential Psychopharmacology: Neuroscientific Basis and Practical Application, 2nd edn.* Cambridge: Cambridge University Press.

Szabadi E. 2006. Drugs for sleep disorders: mechanisms for therapeutic prospects. *Br. J. Clin. Pharmacol.*, 61(6):761–6.

Wang SJ, Yang TT. 2005. Role of central glutamatergic neurotransmission in the pathogenesis of psychiatric and behavioral disorders. *Drug News Perspect.*, 18(9):561–6.

Ziemann U, Meintzschel F, Korchounov A, Ilic TV. 2006. Pharmacological modulation of plasticity in the human motor cortex. *Neurorehabil. Neural Repair*, 20(2): 243–51.

# Basics of prescribing psychopharmacologic agents

3

In most parts of the world children with mental disorders have limited access to qualified child psychiatrists. The diagnosis and management of mental disorders thus mostly falls to the pediatricians and other practitioners providing primary care to children and adolescents.

Drug regulatory processes vary in different countries. In the USA, the regulatory agency is the Food and Drug Administration (FDA). The FDA regulates the safety and efficacy of drugs and the manufacturers' labeling and advertising. An increasingly cautious approach in the use of psychopharmacological agents has been suggested by drug regulatory agencies in recent years. This is exemplified in the USA by the FDA-required labeling of stronger warnings for all FDA-approved medications for attention deficit/hyperactivity disorder (i.e. stimulants, atomoxetine) regarding the potential for sudden cardiac deaths (Box 3.1), and the "black box" warning for all antidepressant medications regarding suicidal potential (Box 3.2).

Although more data are now available for many drugs used in pediatric psychopharmacology, for most the data on long-term safety and efficacy are insufficient. Only a handful of drugs have FDA-approved labeling for use in children and adolescents. Lack of FDA labeling does not necessarily indicate that a drug should not be used or is contraindicated for use in children; it means lack of controlled clinical trials in the pediatric age group to assess a drug's safety and efficacy. Thus, in most cases, the use of psychopharmacologic agents in children and adolescents is considered "off-label." Various medications used in pediatric psychopharmacology are listed in Table 3.1.

49

**Box 3.1.** Warning for cardiovascular risks for US FDA approved drugs for attention deficit/hyperactivity disorder

**Serious cardiovascular events; sudden death and pre-existing structural cardiac abnormalities or other serious heart problems**

Children and adolescents

Sudden death has been reported in association with CNS stimulant treatment at usual doses in children and adolescents with structural cardiac abnormalities or other serious heart problems. Although some serious heart problems alone carry an increased risk of sudden death, stimulant products generally should not be used in children or adolescents with known serious structural cardiac abnormalities, cardiomyopathy, serious heart rhythm abnormalities, or other serious cardiac problems that may place them at increased vulnerability to the sympathomimetic effects of a stimulant drug.

**Adults**

Sudden deaths, stroke, and myocardial infarction have been reported in adults taking stimulant drugs at usual doses for ADHD. Although the role of stimulants in these adult cases is also unknown, adults have a greater likelihood than children of having serious structural cardiac abnormalities, cardiomyopathy, serious heart rhythm abnormalities, coronary artery disease, or other serious cardiac problems. Adults with such abnormalities should also generally not be treated with stimulant drugs.

**Hypertension and other cardiovascular conditions**

Stimulant medications cause a modest increase in average blood pressure (about 2–3 mm Hg) and average heart rate (about 3–6 bpm) and individuals may have larger increases. While the mean changes alone would not be expected to have short-term consequences, all patients should be monitored for larger changes in heart rate and blood pressure. Caution is indicated in treating patients whose underlying medical conditions might be compromised by increase in blood pressure or heart rate, e.g. those with pre-existing hypertension, heart failure, recent myocardial infarction, or ventricular arrhythmia.

**Assessing cardiovascular status in patients being treated with stimulant medications**

Children, adolescents, or adults who are being considered for treatment with stimulant medications, should have a careful history (including assessment for family history of sudden death or ventricular arrhythmia) and physical exam to assess for the presence of cardiac disease, and should receive further evaluation if findings suggest such diseases (e.g. electrocardiogram and echocardiogram). Patients who develop symptoms such as exertional chest pain, unexplained syncope, or other symptoms suggestive of cardiac disease during stimulant treatment should undergo a prompt cardiac evaluation.

Source: www.fda.gov

**Box 3.2.** Black box warning for suicidality risk of antidepressants and atomoxetine

Suicidality in children and adolescents – Antidepressants increased the risk of suicidal thinking and behavior (suicidality) in short-term studies in children and adolescents with major depressive disorder and other psychiatric disorders. Anyone considering the use of [antidepressant name] in a child or adolescent must balance this risk with the clinical need. Patients who are started on therapy should be observed closely for clinical worsening, suicidality, or unusual changes in behavior. Families and caregivers should be advised of the need for close observation and communication with the prescriber.

Pooled analyses of short-term (4 to 16 weeks) placebo-controlled trials of 9 antidepressant drugs (SSRIs and others) in children and adolescents with major depressive disorder, obsessive-compulsive disorder, or other psychiatric disorders (a total of 24 trials involving over 4400 patients) have revealed a greater risk of adverse events representing suicidal thinking or behavior (suicidality) during the first few months of treatment in those receiving antidepressants. The average risk of such events in patients receiving antidepressants was 4%, twice the placebo risk of 2%. No suicides occurred in these trials.

Source: www.fda.gov

As such the prescribing physician must clearly document the rationale for off-label use. There is very little clinical experience and few research data on the use of psychopharmacologic agents in pre-school age children (i.e. 6 years or younger) and expert consultation should be considered before using these agents in this age group. Medicolegal and ethical considerations also pose significant dilemmas in research as well as in the clinical treatment of children with mental disorders. Some practical considerations, useful in prescribing a psychopharmacological agent for children and adolescents, are outlined below.

## ■ Diagnosis

Before considering any pharmacological intervention a clear diagnosis should be established. In addition, specific target symptoms should be identified for treatment.

## ■ History

In addition to the diagnostic history and examination, a thorough history of use of any therapeutic medications, illicit drug use, use of nonprescription

**Table 3.1** Medications used to treat emotional and behavioral problems in children and adolescents, including indications and ages for which use is approved.

| Class | Agent | Indications* | Ages (years) |
|---|---|---|---|
| **Psychostimulants** | | | |
| **Sympathomimetics** | | | |
| Oral: regular release | Methylphenidate (MPH) | ADHD, narcolepsy | $\geq 6$ |
| | Dex-MPH | ADHD | $\geq 6$ |
| | Mixed amphetamines | ADHD; narcolepsy | $\geq 3; \geq 6$ |
| | Dextroamphetamine | ADHD; narcolepsy | $\geq 3; \geq 6$ |
| Oral: extended release | Methylphenidate | ADHD | $\geq 6$ |
| | Dex-MPH | ADHD | $\geq 6$ |
| | Mixed amphetamines | ADHD | $\geq 6$ |
| | Dextroamphetamine | ADHD; narcolepsy | $\geq 3; \geq 6$ |
| Transdermal | Methylphenidate | ADHD | 6–12 |
| **Other** | Modafinil | Narcolepsy, OSAHS; ADHD‡ | $\geq 16$ |
| **Antidepressants** | | | |
| Tricyclics | Imipramine | Depression, enuresis | $\geq 6$ |
| | Nortriptyline | Depression, enuresis | $\geq 6$ |
| | Amitriptyline | Depression | $\geq 9$ |
| | Clomipramine | OCD | $\geq 10$ |
| | Doxepin | Depression | $\geq 18$ |
| MAOIs | Isocarboxazid | Depression | $\geq 16$ |
| | Phenelzine | Depression | $\geq 18$ |
| | Tranylcypromine | Depression | $\geq 18$ |
| | Selegiline (transdermal) | Depression | $\geq 18$ |
| SSRIs | Fluoxetine | OCD; Depression; Bulimia nervosa, Panic disorder | $\geq 7; \geq 8;$ $\geq 18$ |
| | Paroxetine | OCD, Depression, PTSD, GAD, SAD, Panic disorder | $\geq 18$ |
| | Sertraline | OCD; Depression, PTSD, PMDD, SAD, Panic disorder | $\geq 6; \geq 18$ |
| | Fluvoxamine | OCD | $\geq 6$ |
| | Citalopram | Depression | $\geq 18$ |
| | Escitalopram | Depression, GAD | $\geq 18$ |
| SNRIs | Venlafaxine | Depression | $\geq 18$ |
| | Duloxetine | Depression | $\geq 18$ |

**Table 3.1** (*cont.*)

| Class | Agent | Indications* | Ages (years) |
|---|---|---|---|
| Other | Trazodone | Depression | ≥6 |
| | Nefazodone | Depression | ≥18 |
| | Bupropion | Depression; ADHD[‡] | ≥18 |
| | Mirtazapine | Depression | ≥18 |
| | Atomoxetine | ADHD | ≥6 |
| **Antipsychotics** | | | |
| Phenothiazines | Chlorpromazine | Schizophrenia (SCZ); "severe behavioral problems" (SBP) | ≥18; 1–12 |
| | Thioridazine | SCZ; SBP | ≥18; ≥2 |
| Butyrophenones | Haloperidol | SCZ; Tourette's, SBP | ≥18; ≥3 |
| "Atypicals" | Clozapine | SCZ, treatment-resistant | ≥18 |
| | Risperidone | SCZ, BD-I | ≥18 |
| | Olanzapine | SCZ, BD-I | ≥18 |
| | Quetiapine | SCZ, BD-I | ≥18 |
| | Ziprasidone | SCZ, BD-I | ≥18 |
| | Aripiprazole | SCZ, BD-I | ≥18 |
| Other | Pimozide | Tourette's | ≥12 |
| **Mood stabilizers** | | | |
| Lithium salts | Lithium carbonate | BD-I | ≥12 |
| Anticonvulsants | Carbamazepine | Epilepsy; trigeminal neuralgia | Any; ≥18 |
| | Valproic acid | Epilepsy; migraine prophylaxis, BD-I | ≥10; ≥18 |
| | Lamotrigine | Epilepsy; BD-I | ≥2; ≥18 |
| | Oxcarbazepine | Epilepsy | 4–16, ≥18 |
| | Gabapentin | Epilepsy; post-herpetic neuralgia | ≥3; ≥18 |
| | Topiramate | Epilepsy | ≥2 |
| **Alpha-agonists** | Clonidine | Hypertension; ADHD[‡], Tourette's[‡] | ≥12 |
| | Guanfacine | Hypertension; ADHD[‡], Tourette's[‡] | ≥12 |
| **Beta-blockers** | Propranolol^ | Hypertension (all) | ≥18 |
| | Metoprolol | Atrial fibrillation | |
| | Pindolol | Migraine | |

(*cont.*)

**Table 3.1** (*cont.*)

| Class | Agent | Indications* | Ages (years) |
|---|---|---|---|
| | Nadolol | Prophylaxis<br>Essential tremor<br>Aggression‡ (all) | |
| **Anxiolytics** | | | |
| Benzodiazepines | Diazepam | Epilepsy, muscle spasms, anxiety | ≥0.5 |
| | Lorazepam | Anxiety | ≥12 |
| | Clonazepam | Epilepsy; panic disorder | Any; ≥18 |
| Other | Buspirone | Anxiety | ≥6 |

*Abbreviations: ADHD = Attention deficit/hyperactivity disorder; BD-I = Bipolar disorder I; GAD = Generalized anxiety disorder; OCD = Obsessive-compulsive disorder; OSAHS = Obstructive sleep apnea/hypopnea syndrome; SAD = Social anxiety disorder; PMDD = Pre-menstrual dysphoric disorder; PTSD = Post-traumatic stress disorder.

‡ Unapproved indications.

agents, and use of home remedies and herbal remedies should be ascertained. This will have direct implications for drug-drug interactions.

# ■ Psychosocial assessment

Psychosocial factors will have implications for the patient's and parents' or caregivers' ability to adhere to the treatment recommendations. These factors should be explored before a drug regimen is prescribed. Such factors may include the caregiver's education and ability to read, ability to buy the medications, understand how to use them, adequacy of supervision, issues related to access of care, transportation, and other factors.

# ■ Nonpharmacological treatment

Various forms of psychotherapy, psychosocial treatments, and psycho-educational approaches (see Chapter 1) used alone or in combination with pharmacological treatment may be appropriate and must be considered in a comprehensive treatment plan for various mental health disorders in children and adolescents. Pharmacological treatments will not impact the environmental factors that may be contributing to initiating or maintaining the behavioral symptoms and must thus be addressed on their own merit.

# ■ Product information

Once a decision is made to use a drug, it is recommended that the prescribing physician be familiar with or review the manufacturer's complete prescribing or product information, especially indications, contraindications, side effects, recommendations for pretreatment work up, monitoring guidelines, and review any potential drug–drug interactions. Product information can be easily accessed through the manufacturer's website, the FDA website (www.fda.gov), or other drug information resources such as the Physician Desk Reference (www.pdr.com) or epocrates (www.epocrates.com). Other more detailed resources (may be subscription based) for drug information include the AHFS (American Hospital Formulary Service) Drug Information (American Society of Health-System Pharmacists, Bethesda, MD, USA; http://www.ahfsdruginformation.com); and the USP DI Drug Information for the Health Care Professional (Thomson MICOMEDEX, the United States Pharmacoeial Convention, Inc., Greenwood Village, CO, USA; http://www.micomedex.com); and www.lexi.com.

# ■ Informed consent

Informed consent should be obtained and documented in the patient's medical record before initiation of the drug treatment. In older children (generally above age 7 years) and adolescents, *assent* should be obtained and documented. Informed consent should be viewed as an ongoing and dynamic process and should be periodically reviewed in light of emergent therapeutic or adverse effects of the drug as well as adherence issues. Informed consent should include the indication for use, benefits of the drug, side effects or risks of drug use, alternative treatments, and consequences of not using the drug treatment.

# ■ Patient and family education

Key elements of the patient and the family education about the drug treatment include information about such issues as how long it will take before therapeutic effects might be seen, need for clinical (and laboratory if indicated) monitoring, importance of adherence to the treatment plan, or what signs or symptoms to watch for to detect significant treatment emergent adverse reactions. Medication guides providing information on how to use the drug and side effects, written for the patient or caregiver use have been developed by various agencies. In the USA the FDA may require distribution of such medication information guides to the patient at the time the drug is prescribed or dispensed, when there is a serious and significant health concern associated with the use of the drug. In case of antidepressants the US FDA approved product label requires that a medication guide (see example in Appendix 3.1) be given to the patient or the caregiver at the time of dispensing the drug. For therapeutic success it is important to engage the patient and the family in the treatment plan. The instructions to the child or the adolescent should be age and developmentally appropriate.

# ■ Prescription

An appropriate dosage form should be chosen based on such factors as patient preference, cost, availability, and indication. Review the instructions on how to administer the drug (e.g. some drugs should not be crushed, others not mixed, etc.). Many factors affect the appropriate dose for an individual child, as reviewed in Chapter 2; therefore it is prudent to start at the lower end of the dosage range, titrating the dose gradually to achieve the desired therapeutic effects. It may take from several days to several weeks before the optimum therapeutic dose is reached, and several more weeks to months to realize the full therapeutic effects of the drug. Hence, once the optimum dose is reached the patient should be maintained at that level for an appropriate duration. Premature discontinuation or switching of medication is unwise and a common reason for apparent therapeutic failure.

# ■ Switching, augmentation, combination

After an adequate trial of a drug, some patients will be judged to be non-responders and may need to try another agent in the same or a different class. In some patients addition of a second agent, generally of a different class, may augment the partial response to the initial drug. Comorbidity is common in most mental disorders often requiring combination drug therapy. The identification of several different target symptoms may also dictate combination therapy.

## ■ Discontinuation

After an adequate drug trial and other treatments, the disorder may remit and a careful consideration should be given to discontinue the drug. In most cases this should be a gradual process with close monitoring for emergent symptoms. If any symptoms reappear the patient should be put back on the full dose of the drug. Symptoms of discontinuation syndrome that result from abruptly discontinuing the drug should be differentiated from the symptoms of recurrence of the underlying mental disorder.

## ■ Follow-up and monitoring

A long-term plan for regular clinical and – if indicated – laboratory follow-up and monitoring should be reviewed with the family at the time of initiating the drug treatment and during follow-up visits set up well in advance. Adherence to the recommended plan must be emphasized.

## ■ Summary

The research data on most psychopharmacological agents used in children and adolescents are still limited (with the exception of stimulants) while there is evidence of increased use of these agents in children and adolescents. Since access to child and adolescent psychiatrists may be limited in many parts of the world other medical practitioners taking care of children and adolescents manage many of these mental health problems. It is essential to understand some of the basic aspects of prescribing a psychopharmacologic agent.

## ■ Appendix 3.1. Medication guide about using antidepressants in children and teenagers

### What is the most important information I should know if my child is being prescribed an antidepressant?

Parents or guardians need to think about four important things when their child is prescribed an antidepressant:

(1) There is a risk of suicidal thoughts or actions.

(2) How to try to prevent suicidal thoughts or actions in your child.

(3) You should watch for certain signs if your child is taking an antidepressant.

(4) There are benefits and risks when using antidepressants.

## (1)  There is a risk of suicidal thoughts or actions

Children and teenagers sometimes think about suicide, and many report trying to kill themselves.

Antidepressants increase suicidal thoughts and actions in some children and teenagers. But suicidal thoughts and actions can also be caused by depression, a serious medical condition that is commonly treated with antidepressants. Thinking about killing yourself or trying to kill yourself is called *suicidality* or *being suicidal*.

A large study combined the results of 24 different studies of children and teenagers with depression or other illnesses. In these studies, patients took either a placebo (sugar pill) or an antidepressant for 1 to 4 months. *No one committed suicide in these studies*, but some patients became suicidal. On sugar pills, 2 out of every 100 became suicidal. On the antidepressants, 4 out of every 100 patients became suicidal.

For some children and teenagers, the risks of suicidal actions may be especially high. These include patients with:

• Bipolar illness (sometimes called manic-depressive illness).

• A family history of bipolar illness.

• A personal or family history of attempting suicide.

If any of these are present, make sure you tell your healthcare provider before your child takes an antidepressant.

## (2)  How to try to prevent suicidal thoughts and actions

To try to prevent suicidal thoughts and actions in your child, pay close attention to changes in her or his moods or actions, especially if the changes occur suddenly. Other important people in your child's life can help by paying attention as well (e.g. your child, brothers and sisters, teachers, and other important people). The changes to look out for are listed in Section 3, on what to watch for.

Whenever an antidepressant is started or its dose is changed, pay close attention to your child. After starting an antidepressant, your child should generally see his or her healthcare provider:

- Once a week for the first 4 weeks.
- Every 2 weeks for the next 4 weeks.
- After taking the antidepressant for 12 weeks.
- After 12 weeks, follow your healthcare provider's advice about how often to come back.
- More often if problems or questions arise (see Section 3).

You should call your child's healthcare provider between visits if needed.

## (3)  You should watch for certain signs if your child is taking an antidepressant

Contact your child's healthcare provider *right away* if your child exhibits any of the following signs for the first time, or if they seem worse, or worry you, your child, or your child's teacher:

- Thoughts about suicide or dying.
- Attempts to commit suicide.
- New or worse depression.
- New or worse anxiety.
- Feeling very agitated or restless.
- Panic attacks.
- Difficulty sleeping (insomnia).
- New or worse irritability.
- Acting aggressive, being angry, or violent.
- Acting on dangerous impulses.
- An extreme increase in activity and talking.
- Other unusual changes in behavior or mood.

Never let your child stop taking an antidepressant without first talking to his or her healthcare provider. Stopping an antidepressant suddenly can cause other symptoms.

## (4)  There are benefits and risks when using antidepressants

Antidepressants are used to treat depression and other illnesses. Depression and other illnesses can lead to suicide. In some children and teenagers, treatment with an antidepressant increases suicidal thinking or actions. It is important to discuss all the risks of treating depression and also the risks of not treating it. You and your child should discuss all treatment choices with your healthcare provider, not just the use of antidepressants.

Other side effects can occur with antidepressants (see section below).

Of all the antidepressants, only fluoxetine (Prozac™) has been FDA approved to treat pediatric depression.

For obsessive–compulsive disorder in children and teenagers, the FDA has approved only fluoxetine (Prozac™), sertraline (Zoloft™), fluvoxamine, and clomipramine (Anafranil™). [Prozac® is a registered trademark of Eli Lilly and Company; Zoloft® is a registered trademark of Pfizer Pharmaceuticals; Anafranil® is a registered trademark of Mallinckrodt Inc.]

Your healthcare provider may suggest other antidepressants based on the past experience of your child or other family members.

## ■ Is this all I need to know if my child is being prescribed an antidepressant?

No. This is a warning about the risk for suicidality. Other side effects can occur with antidepressants. Be sure to ask your healthcare provider to explain all the side effects of the particular drug he or she is prescribing. Also ask about drugs to avoid when taking an antidepressant. Ask your healthcare provider or pharmacist where to find more information.

[This medication guide has been approved by the U.S. Food and Drug Administration for all antidepressants. Revised 1/26/05.]

SELECTED BIBLIOGRAPHY

Nissen SE. 2006. ADHD drugs and cardiovascular risk. *N. Engl. J. Med.*, 354:1445.

Ryan ND. 2005. Treatment of depression in children and adolescents. *Lancet*, 366: 933–40.

Thomson Healthcare. 2007. *Physicians' Desk Reference, 61st edition*. Montvale, NJ: Thomson Healthcare.

United Kingdom Drug Regulation Agency: Medicines and Healthcare Products Regulatory Agency, Department of Health, UK. http://www.mhra.gov.uk

United States Drug Regulatory Agency: Food and Drug Administration. http://www.fda.gov

Whittington CJ, Kendall T, Fonagy P, Cottrell D, Cotgrove A, Boddington E. 2004. Selective serotonin reuptake inhibitors in childhood depression: systematic review of published versus unpublished data. *Lancet*, 363:1341–5.

# Anxiety disorders

4

## ■ Definition

*Anxiety* is characterized by an apprehensive anticipation or fear by the child or adolescent of some dangerous occurrence in the future. Anxiety is usually accompanied by unpleasant feelings, stress or tension and somatic symptoms and signs. *Anxiety disorder* is characterized by persistent fear or worry that causes significant distress and impairment of age-appropriate functioning such as school work, play, and interpersonal relations. The symptoms in anxiety disorder take up a significant amount of daily time of the child or the adolescent and such symptoms last over a period of several months, typically 6 or more months. Types of specific anxiety disorders as classified in the DSM–IV–TR are listed in Table 4.1.

## ■ Epidemiology

Anxiety disorders are highly prevalent in children and adolescents. The etiological theories implicate genetic factors, temperamental characteristics of the child, and environmental risk factors. The prevalence rate of anxiety disorders in children has been reported to be between 6% and 20%. The prevalence has been reported to be between 0.3% and 13% in the pre-adolescent age and between 0.6% and 7% in the adolescent age group. Some studies suggest that anxiety disorders may be more common in girls compared with boys. The age of onset varies depending on the specific disorder. Although the long-term course of childhood anxiety disorders is not clearly delineated, it is generally recognized that most tend to persist into adulthood. Adolescents with anxiety disorders are at a significantly higher risk for substance use, particularly alcohol use. The long-term psychosocial impact of anxiety disorders is significant. Anxiety disorders also have a high rate of other comorbid mental health disorders.

**Table 4.1** DSM–IV–TR classification of anxiety disorders.

Panic disorder without agoraphobia
Agoraphobia without history of panic disorder
Specific phobia
Social phobia
Obsessive-compulsive disorder
Posttraumatic stress disorder
Acute stress disorder
Generalized anxiety disorder
Anxiety disorder due to a general medical condition
Substance-induced anxiety disorder
Anxiety disorder not otherwise specified
Separation anxiety disorder

**Table 4.2** Differential diagnoses of anxiety disorders.

Agoraphobia
Anxiety disorder due to general medical condition
Anxiety disorder not otherwise specified
Acute stress disorder
Adjustment disorder with anxious mood
Childhood developmental fears and phobias
Competitive anxiety in athletes
Generalized anxiety disorder
Hyperventilation
Hypochondriasis
Obsessive-compulsive disorder
Panic attacks and panic disorder
Posttraumatic stress disorder
Selective mutism
Separation anxiety disorder
Social phobia
Somatization disorder
Specific phobia
Substance-induced anxiety disorder

# ■ Differential diagnoses/comorbid disorders

Conditions that should be considered in the differential diagnoses of anxiety disorders are listed in Table 4.2 and conditions comorbid with anxiety disorders are listed in conditions in Table 4.3. Symptoms of anxiety or anxiety

**Table 4.3** Mental health disorders comorbid with anxiety disorders.

Major depressive disorder (most common)
Other mood disorders
Attention deficit/hyperactivity disorder
Oppositional defiant disorder
Conduct disorder
Learning disorders
Language disorders

**Table 4.4** Selected conditions with clinically significant anxiety symptoms/disorders.

*Genetic syndromes*
Down syndrome
Fragile X syndrome
Neurofibromatosis type 1
Prader–Willi syndrome
Velocardiofacial syndrome

*Medical conditions*
Epilepsy
Fetal alcohol syndrome
Hyperthyroidism
Hyperparathyroidism
Hyperadrenocorticism
Hypoglycemia
Mitral valve prolapse
Pheochromocytoma
Porphyria
Vestibular dysfunction

disorders are also a significant clinical feature of certain genetic and medical conditions as listed in Table 4.4.

Normal developmental fears that vary depending upon the age and developmental stage of the child should not be confused with anxiety disorders. Infants may be fearful of sudden loud noises and strangers; the preschool child may have fear of animals, the dark, imaginary creatures or the storms. Anticipatory anxiety may first manifest during preschool age. The school-age child may have fears related to attending the school such as acceptance by peers at school, about a particular subject or teacher. During the adolescent years fears may be of the future events, about one's physical appearance, and sexuality.

# ■ Psychopharmacology

## Medication classification and mechanism of action

Some of the medications more commonly used in practice to treat various anxiety symptoms and disorders are listed in Table 4.5.

(1) Selective serotonin reuptake inhibitors (SSRIs): SSRIs block the reuptake of serotonin into presynaptic neurons and enhance serotonergic neurotransmission.

(2) Serotonin and Norepinephrine Reuptake Inhibitors (SNRIs): Duloxetine and venlafaxine block both the serotonin and norepinephrine reuptake and increase serotonergic, noradrenergic, and dopaminergic neurotransmission.

(3) Tricyclic antidepressants (TCAs): The TCAs block the reuptake to a varying degree of the monoamine neurotransmitters (dopamine, norepinephrine, and serotonin) into the presynaptic neurons. TCAs also have significant anticholinergic and antihistaminic effects.

(4) Benzodiazepines (BDZs): BDZs bind to the benzodiazepine receptors in the CNS at the gamma aminobutyric acid-A (GABA-A) ligand-gated chloride channel complex and enhance the inhibitory effects of GABA. Benzodiazepines facilitate the chloride conductance through GABA-regulated channels. Their therapeutic effects in reducing anxiety symptoms are believed to be due to inhibition of amygdala-centered neuronal circuits.

(5) Other: *Buspirone* is an azapirone and a serotonin 1A partial agonist. The anxiolytic effects of buspirone are believed to be due to its postsynaptic partial agonist actions reducing serotonergic activity. *Hydroxyzine* is an antihistamine and it acts by blocking the histamine 1 receptors. *Nefazodone* is a SARI (serotonin 2 antagonist/reuptake inhibitor) antidepressant and works via antagonism at the postsynaptic serotonin 5-HT receptor; it also blocks presynaptic serotonin reuptake. *Mirtazepine* is an antagonist of the pre-synaptic norepinephrine alpha 2 receptor; it also blocks postsynaptic 5-HT2 and 5-HT3 receptors.

    *Propranolol* is a beta-blocker. It blocks the beta-adrenergic receptors, effectively reducing sympathetic nervous system activity. It is not known how beta-blockers exert their effects on the CNS, as agents vary by degree and selectivity for beta 1 (mostly cardiac) and beta 2 (noncardiac) receptors, and also vary in degree of lipophilicity.

**Table 4.5** Medications used in anxiety disorders.

| Class | Agent | Dosing Initial (mg) | Dosing Daily range (mg) and schedule | Ages[a] and anxiety disorders |
|---|---|---|---|---|
| *Antidepressants* | | | | |
| SSRIs | Citalopram | 5–20 | 10–60 qd | NA |
| | Escitalopram | 1.25–5 | 2.5–20 qd | ≥ 18 GAD |
| | Fluvoxamine | 12.5–50 | 50–300 qd-bid | ≥ 6 OCD |
| | Fluoxetine | 5–20 | 10–80 qd | ≥ 7 OCD |
| | Sertraline | 12.5–25 | 50–200 qd-bid | ≥ 6 OCD |
| | | | | ≥ 18 PD, SAD, PTSD |
| SNRIs | Duloxetine | 20 | 40–60 bid | NA |
| | Venlafaxine | 12.5–37.5 | 25–300 bid | ≥ 18 PD, SAD, GAD |
| TCAs | Clomipramine | 12.5–25 | 2–5 mg/kg/d qhs-bid | ≥ 10 OCD |
| | Imipramine | 10–25 | 2–5 mg/kg/d qhs-bid | NA |
| | Nortriptyline | 10 | 1–3 mg/kg/d qhs-bid | NA |
| | Protriptyline | 5–10 | 0.5–2 mg/kg/d bid-qid | NA |
| Others | Nefazodone | 25–50 | 25–400 qhs-bid | NA |
| | Mirtazepine | 7.5–15 | 15–45 qhs | NA |
| *Anxiolytics* | | | | |
| Benzodiazepines | Alprazolam | 0.125 | 1–6 tid-qid | ≥ 18 GAD, PD |
| | Chlordiazepoxide | 2.5–5 | 15–40 tid-qid | ≥ 18 any |
| | Clonazepam | 0.125–0.5 | 0.125–3 qhs-bid | ≥ 18 PD |
| | Diazepam | 1–2 | 0.5–4 qhs-bid | ≥ 0.5 any |
| | Lorazepam | 0.125–0.5 | 0.125–4 qhs-bid | ≥ 12 any |
| Others | Buspirone | 2.5 | 5–60 bid-tid | ≥ 18 any |
| | Hydroxyzine | 12.5–25 | 50–100 bid-qid | Any[b] |
| | Propranolol | 10–20 | 20–40 bid | NA |

[a] Ages (years) are for FDA-approved indications (see Table 3.1, Chapter 3, for details); use for other indications and/or at other ages is based on clinical judgement.

[b] No minimum age specified; can be used for "anxiety and tension."

SSRIs, selective serotonin reuptake inhibitors; SNRIs, serotonin-norepinephrine reuptake inhibitors; TCAs, tricyclic antidepressants; GAD, generalized anxiety disorder; OCD, obsessive-compulsive disorder; PD, panic disorder; PTSD, post-traumatic stress disorder; SAD, social anxiety disorder; NA, not approved for anxiety disorders.

## Dosages

Dosages for most medications used in the pediatric age group are not fully established and it is prudent to start at the lower end of the dosage range and to slowly titrate the dose to achieve therapeutic effect. Typical dosages used in the pediatric anxiety disorders are listed in Table 4.5.

## Side effects

### Selective serotonin reuptake inhibitors

The common side effects of the SSRIs are nausea, decreased appetite, dry mouth, increased sweating, insomnia, headaches, diarrhea, rash, nervousness, agitation, and akathisia. SSRIs also cause sexual dysfunction both in males and females. Sexual side effects include delayed orgasm, anorgasmia, and decreased libido. Most of these nonlife threatening side effects tend to diminish with time. Mammoplasia in girls and gynecomastia in boys have also been reported.

SSRIs can alter the sleep architecture. SSRIs can reduce the total duration of sleep and the duration of rapid-eye-movement sleep. Sleep disturbances are common in patients taking SSRIs and include difficulty falling or staying asleep, daytime drowsiness, and vivid and frightening dreams.

Some patients on SSRIs (and antidepressant medications in general) may experience *behavioral activation*. Behavioral activation is much more common in children and adolescents when compared with adults and reported incidence ranges from 20–50%. Activation is more common during the initial days and weeks of starting the SSRI and after an increase in dose. Behavioral activation is characterized by alteration in mood, dysphoria, altered cognition, nervousness, agitation, irritability, and in severe cases by akathisia (uncomfortable sensation of restlessness that can be physical or psychological or both). Although hypomania, mania, and acute psychotic reactions have also been reported, behavioral activation is neither an indication of nor predictive of bipolar disorder. Some of the symptoms seen in behavioral activation overlap those of discontinuation syndrome and a careful history of adherence to medication regimen should be ascertained to differentiate the two conditions.

In contrast to activation in which the mood state remains the same, *switching* (or *bipolar switching*) is characterized by treatment-emergent change in mood state from depressed mood to mania or hypomania in patients taking SSRIs (and other antidepressants). The patient and the family recognize these as new symptoms not present before the treatment was started with an SSRI agent. Switching is a less common but significant side effect of SSRIs in children and adolescents. Bipolar switching should be differentiated from behavioral activation. Symptoms of switching tend to occur later in the course of the treatment and may not abate even after discontinuation of the SSRI agent. Development of symptoms suggestive of bipolar disorder requires discontinuation of SSRIs and starting appropriate treatment for bipolar disorder after further evaluation (see Chapter 6). Children and adolescents when effectively treated for anxiety or depression with an SSRI agent may also then manifest symptoms of comorbid disorders more clearly (e.g. symptoms of attention deficit/hyperactivity disorder or conduct disorder).

A more serious adverse event associated with SSRIs is the *central serotonin syndrome* (CSS), which is caused by excessive central nervous system serotonergic activity. Although CSS, can occur when the patient is on a single SSRI agent at high doses, it is potentially more likely to occur when the patient is on multiple SSRIs or other agents with serotonergic effects (Table 4.6).

Central serotonin syndrome is characterized by agitation, confusion, tachycardia, hypo- or hypertension, resting tremors, incoordination, muscular rigidity, myoclonus, hyperreflexia, fever, shivering, excessive sweating, diaphoresis, and diarrhea. Central serotonin syndrome can result in seizures, metabolic acidosis, rhabdomyolysis, disseminated intravascular coagulation, respiratory failure, coma, and death. When CSS is suspected, all serotonergic medications must be discontinued and immediate general medical care must be initiated including inpatient care and appropriate consultations.

*Discontinuation syndrome* has been described with abrupt discontinuation of an SSRI agent after several weeks of use, characterized by dysphoric mood, irritability, agitation, dizziness, sensory disturbances (e.g. electric shock-like sensations), anxiety, tearfulness, confusion, nightmares, and sleep disturbances. For most SSRIs, symptoms are seen within 1–3 days of reducing the dose or discontinuation of the medication; in the case of fluoxetine, because of its longer half life, symptoms of discontinuation may not be seen until after 7–10 days of stopping the medication. Most symptoms associated with discontinuation of SSRI agents generally resolve within 1–2 weeks. Sometimes severe symptoms associated with discontinuation of

**Table 4.6** High-risk drugs for central serotonin syndrome.

| Class | Examples |
| --- | --- |
| SSRIs | Citalopram |
| | Escitalopram |
| | Fluvoxamine |
| | Fluoxetine |
| | Sertraline |
| | Paroxetine |
| SNRIs | Venlafaxine |
| TCAs | Imipramine |
| | Clomipramine |
| | Amitriptyline |
| MAOIs | Selegiline |
| | Phenelzine |
| | Tranylcypromine |
| Other | Buspirone |
| | Nefazodone |
| | Trazodone |
| Antipsychotics | Risperidone |
| | Olanzapine |
| | Quetiapine |
| Mood stabilizers | Lithium |
| Antimigraine agents | Sumatriptan |
| | Dihydroergotamine |
| Other | L-tryptophan |
| | Amphetamines |
| | Cocaine |
| | MDMA |
| | LSD |
| | Dextromethorphan |

SSRIs, selective serotonin reuptake inhibitors; SNRIs, serotonin-norepinephrine reuptake inhibitors; TCAs, tricyclic antidepressants; MAOIs, mono-amine oxidase inhibitors.

an SSRI agent may require restarting the patient on an SSRI at a lower dose for a short period and gradually tapering the medication. Symptoms of discontinuation syndrome should be differentiated from those of recurrence of anxiety disorder.

Apathy or amotivational syndrome, extrapyramidal symptoms, and increased bleeding tendencies including gastrointestinal bleeding have been reported in pediatric patients on SSRIs. There is an increased risk of adverse events with the use of SSRIs in patients who are significantly underweight, have underlying hepatic or renal disease, have a history of atrial tachycardia or conduction disorders, and those who have a history of excessive daytime sleepiness.

The issue of *suicidality* with the use of SSRIs and other antidepressants in the treatment of depression is discussed in Chapter 6 (also see Box 3.2, Chapter 3).

## Serotonin and norepinephrine reuptake inhibitors

Duloxetine and venlafaxine have largely similar side effects as those of SSRIs, in addition to more significant increase in systemic blood pressure. Hyponatremia and syndrome of inappropriate antidiuretic hormone secretion are uncommon but significant side effects reported with the use of venlafaxine.

## Tricyclic antidepressants

The effects that the tricyclic antidepressants (TCAs) can have on the cardiovascular system can range from mild tachycardia and hypotension to cardiac arrhythmia, prolongation of PR interval, QRS, QTc, and heart blocks. The cardiovascular side effects are dose related. The use of desipramine in children has been associated with some sudden cardiac deaths.

Other side effects include dry mouth, blurred vision, constipation, diarrhea, urinary retention, increased appetite, unusual taste in mouth, weight gain, heart burn, increased fatigue, dizziness, sedation, hyperprolactinemia, and hypoglycemia or hyperglycemia. Uncommon but significant side effects include dilutional hyponatremia, lowered seizure threshold, increased intraocular pressure, and hepatotoxicity. (Side effects of TCAs are listed in Chapter 5, Table 5.13.)

## Benzodiazepines

Side effects of BZDs include sedation, cognitive blunting, dizziness, ataxia, nystagmus, bradycardia, transitory hallucinations, memory impairment (typically anterograde amnesia), constipation, diplopia, hypotension, urinary incontinence or retention, fatigue, slurred speech, paradoxical hyperexcitability, and nervousness. Higher dose and longer duration of treatment increase the risk of side effects. Benzodiazepines are potentially habit forming and can lead to addiction and dependence. Less common but significant and potentially life-threatening side-effects include: respiratory depression, hepatotoxicity, renal dysfunction, and blood dyscrasias.

## Other medication

Side effects of buspirone are generally mild and include headache, dizziness, nervousness, sedation, nausea, lightheadedness, restlessness, and excitement. Hydroxyzine may cause dry mouth, sedation, tremor, increased appetite, and constipation.

Mirtazepine is quite sedating (especially at lower doses), frequently causes weight gain, may elevate serum cholesterol and transaminases, and may impair cognition. Other side effects of mirtazepine include dry mouth, constipation, dizziness, abnormal dreams, confusion, nausea, blurred vision, orthostatic hypotension, and flu-like symptoms.

A potentially serious side effect of nefazodone is unpredictable acute hepatic failure. Other side effects of nefazodone include nausea, dry mouth, constipation, dyspepsia, increased appetite and weight gain, headaches, dizziness, insomnia, agitation, confusion, memory impairment, increased cough, priapism, and postural hypotension.

Common side effects of propranolol include dizziness, fatigue, bradycardia, mental status change, gastrointestinal upset, and various skin rashes. Less common but more serious adverse events associated with propranolol use include bronchospasm and heart failure, both of which may occur more readily in children. It is also associated with Raynaud's phenomenon in some patients.

## Contraindications

### Selective serotonin reuptake inhibitors

As a class, the SSRIs should not be used concomitantly with MAOIs, pimozide, or triptans. In addition, neither fluoxetine nor paroxetine should be used with thioridazine. The SSRIs should be used with extreme caution if other serotonergic agents are also being used (Table 4.6). Some of the drug interactions associated with SSRIs are listed in Table 4.7.

### Serotonin and norepinephrine reuptake inhibitors

Duloxetine and venlafaxine have similar precautions and contraindications as those of SSRIs. History of hypertension and other cardiovascular

**Table 4.7** Selected SSRI-drug interactions.

| | |
|---|---|
| SSRI increase the levels of | Phenytoin |
| | TCAs |
| | Nefazodone |
| SSRI may increase or decrease the level of | Lithium |
| SSRI may decrease the level of | Buspirone |
| SSRI level increased by | Cimetidine |
| | MAOIs |
| | Methylphenidate |
| | Phenothiazines |
| SSRI level decreased by | Carbamazepine |
| | Barbiturates |

SSRIs, selective serotonin reuptake inhibitors; TCAs, tricyclic
antidepressants; MAOIs, mono-amine oxidase inhibitors.

disorders may preclude use of SNRIs. These agents should be used with
great caution in patients with a history of seizures.

## Tricyclic antidepressants

The TCAs should not be used concomitantly with the MAOIs, or with medications that are associated with cardiac conduction disorders. They should
be used with caution in patients with a history of seizures, narrow-angle
glaucoma, or those who are on thyroid supplementation. Tricyclic antidepressants are contraindicated in patients with known cardiac disease and
combination of a TCA and clonidine should be avoided because of significant increased risk of hypertension.

## Benzodiazepines

Benzodiazepines should not be used in patients with narrow angle glaucoma. Abuse or dependence potential may exclude use in some patients.
The safety and efficacy of BZDs in the long-term treatment of anxiety disorders in children and adolescents have not been established.

## Other medication

Buspirone should not be used with MAOIs; certain SSRIs used concomitantly with buspirone may reduce its clearance and raise its plasma levels. Carbamazepine increases the clearance of buspirone. Buspirone will

increase the plasma levels of haloperidol. Hydroxyzine will potentiate the effects of another CNS depressant used concomitantly. Do not use mirtazepine with MAOIs. Use mirtazepine with caution in patients with a history of epilepsy. Nefazodone should not be used with carbamazepine, pimozide, or MAOIs. In addition, nefazodone should not be used in patients with hepatic dysfunction.

The major contraindications to propranolol use pertain to the cardiovascular and respiratory systems. The beta blockers should not be used in patients with sinus bradycardia and greater than first-degree heart block, asthma, sick sinus syndrome, significant peripheral arterial disease, pheochromocytoma, insulin-dependent diabetes mellitus, hyperthyroidism, and right ventricular failure associated with pulmonary hypertension.

## How to use the medications

### Selective serotonin reuptake inhibitors

SSRIs are the first line of treatment for treatment of anxiety disorders in children and adolescents. Several well-controlled studies have provided evidence of their safety and effectiveness in the treatment of anxiety disorders in children and adolescents. Studies suggest that treatment of anxiety disorders may require dosages that are relatively higher to those compared with their use in the treatment of depression and the response may take longer. There is no conclusive evidence that suggests superiority of one SSRI over another, and no long-term studies are available to guide the decision for duration of treatment. At least 12 months of use is recommended before trial off the medication; if there is a recurrence of symptoms, the patient should be placed back on the medication.

Once treatment is initiated, the agent should be continued for at least 4 weeks before a decision is made either to increase the dose or to switch to a different SSRI. Dosage increase should occur no less frequently than every 4 weeks. The medication is increased until positive clinical response is obtained, intolerable (or dangerous) side effects emerge, or a maximum dosage has been reached with no or inadequate clinical response. Due to higher rate of drug metabolism in children and adolescents, dosing of certain medications that are typically given once daily in adults may have to be divided into twice daily dosing to prevent withdrawal effects. The safety and efficacy of medications other than SSRIs in the treatment of children and adolescent with anxiety disorders are not fully established at the present time.

## Serotonin and Norepinephrine reuptake inhibitors

Duloxetine and venlafaxine are not considered as first-line treatment for pediatric anxiety disorders. Venlafaxine has been used in some cases as a second choice in those who have failed adequate trial of SSRI. There no clinical trial or experience with use of duloxetine in pediatric anxiety disorders.

## Tricyclic antidepressants

Tricyclic antidepressants are not the preferred drugs for treatment of anxiety disorders in children and adolescents. Tricyclic antidepressants should be started at a low dosage and titrated slowly, monitoring the patient's clinical status, drug plasma levels, and the ECG (the latter being more important than the drug plasma level). Toxicity may occur even if the plasma drug level is in the therapeutic range (see Chapter 6, Table 6.4), so monitoring of the ECG for prolongation of PR, QRS, and $QT_c$ is important. The use of desipramine is generally not recommended in children because of its unfavorable risk–benefit ratio.

## Benzodiazepines

Benzodiazepines have not been shown to be efficacious in the long-term treatment of anxiety disorders in children and adolescents. Their use is limited to short-term treatment in patients with severe anxiety symptoms for rapid effects before the effects of psychotherapy and/or SSRIs can be achieved. Benzodiazepines are often used for procedure-related anxiety.

## Other medication

Buspirone has a high safety profile and may be considered as one of the first-line treatments for anxiety disorders after SSRIs. Buspirone is not associated with dependence or addiction risks and can be used as an augmenting agent to treat anxiety.

Hydroxyzine is not useful for long-term treatment of anxiety disorders in children and adolescents. Its main use is for short-term effects in special circumstances in patients with anxiety symptoms associated with organic diseases, pre-medication for sedation, anxiety, and pruritis associated with allergic conditions, acute hysteria, and anxiety associated with alcohol withdrawal.

Mirtazepine and nefazodone may be considered as the last choice in the treatment of pediatric anxiety disorders in refractory patients. Propranolol is often used to reduce anxiety and tremors associated with certain specific situations such as performance anxiety and acute anxiety in athletes in competitive sports. Although propranolol and other beta-blockers have been shown to be efficacious in ameliorating symptoms of anxiety in adults, especially somatic symptoms of anxiety, no controlled studies support their use in the treatment of anxiety disorders in children and adolescents.

## How to monitor the medications

### Selective serotonin reuptake inhibitors

In patients on SSRIs no specific laboratory monitoring is indicated. Patients should be monitored clinically for side effects. In patients being treated with antidepressants such as SSRIs and TCAs careful clinical monitoring for potential increased risk for suicidal behaviors is recommended. The current US FDA labeling suggests that the patient who is started on an antidepressant be seen by the physician (face to face) once a week for the first 4 weeks of the treatment; biweekly for the second month of treatment; and at the end of the 12th week on medication; however most experts favor an individualized approach that takes into consideration the unique needs and circumstances of the patient and his or her family.

### Serotonin and norepinephrine reuptake inhibitors

In addition to the monitoring guidelines noted for SSRIs, blood pressure should be routinely monitored in patients on SNRIs and blood cholesterol and lipid profile should be checked periodically.

### Tricyclic antidepressants

An ECG should be obtained at baseline, during dosage titration, and after subsequent increases in dosage. The baseline acceptable values for ECG measures recommended by the American Heart Association are: PR interval $\leq 200$ ms; QRS $\leq 120$ ms; and $QT_c \leq 460$ ms. Check blood glucose and serum sodium levels periodically. Check serum prolactin if gynecomastia or menstrual irregularities appear. Check liver function tests if unexplained gastrointestinal symptoms are present.

## Benzodiazepines

For patients on long-term therapy periodic blood testing for completed blood count (to check for neutropenia) and liver function tests (to check for elevated bilirubin or LDH) are suggested.

## Other medication

No laboratory monitoring is indicated with the use of buspirone or hydroxyzine. Although no specific laboratory tests are recommended for mirtazepine and nefazodone use, in younger patients it is prudent to periodically check serum cholesterol, lipid profile, complete blood count, liver function tests, and closely monitor weight gain, body mass index, and blood glucose.

For patients on propranolol, blood pressure and heart rate should be routinely monitored to detect a significant drop in heart rate from baseline. A baseline ECG is also recommended to detect asymptomatic cardiac conduction abnormalities. Before starting propranolol, fasting blood glucose should be obtained. Propranolol can sometimes cause elevations in serum potassium, AST, ALT, and alkaline phosphatase in hypertensive patients.

## ■ Summary

A multimodal approach that integrates psychotherapy (especially exposure-based cognitive-behavior therapy, see Table 1.2 in Chapter 1), family and patient education, and use of medication (mostly an SSRI) if indicated is recommended for pediatric anxiety disorders. In those patients who might benefit from use of medications, SSRIs are the treatment of choice and should be considered in patients with moderate to severe symptoms that may make participation in psychotherapy difficult or in patients whose response to psychotherapy is considered to be inadequate especially in terms of improving functional impairment. Comorbid disorders must be recognized and appropriately and adequately treated at the same time. The response to treatment varies depending upon the severity and specific type of the anxiety disorder and range from 50% to more than 70%. Recurrence of the same, or development of a different type of anxiety disorder, is not uncommon and in most patients, anxiety disorders tend to persist into adulthood requiring long-term treatment planning.

# SELECTED BIBLIOGRAPHY

American Academy of Child and Adolescent Psychiatry. 2007. Practice parameter for the assessment and treatment of children and adolescents with anxiety disorders. *J. Am. Acad. Child Adolescent Psychiatry*, 46(2):267–83.

Baldwin DS, Anderson IM, Nutt DJ *et al.* 2005. Evidence-based guidelines for the pharmacological treatment of anxiety disorders: recommendations from the British Association for Psychopharmacology. *J. Psychopharmacol.*, 19(6):567–96.

Coyle JT. 2001. Drug treatment of anxiety disorders in children. *N. Engl. J. Med.*, 34:1326–7.

Fisher PH, Tobkes JL, Kotcher L, Masia-Warner C. 2006. Psychosocial and pharmacological treatment for pediatric anxiety disorders. *Expert Rev. Neurother.*, 6(11):1707–19.

Hammerness PG, Vivas FM, Geller DA. 2005. Selective serotonin reuptake inhibitors in pediatric psychopharmacology: a review of the evidence. *J. Pediatrics*, 148:158–65.

Kapczinski F, Lima MS, Souza JS, Schmitt R. 2003. Antidepressants for generalized anxiety disorder. *Cochrane Database Syst Rev.*, (2):CD003592.

O'Kearney RT, Anstey KJ, von Sanden C. 2006. Behavioural and cognitive behavioural therapy for obsessive compulsive disorder in children and adolescents. *Cochrane Database Syst. Rev.*, 18(4):CD004856.

Pine DS. 2002. Treating children and adolescents with selective serotonin reuptake inhibitors: how long is appropriate? *J. Child Adolesc. Psychopharmacol.*, 12(3):189–203.

Reinblatt SP, Walkup JT. 2005. Psychopharmacologic treatment of pediatric anxiety disorders. *Child Adolesc. Psychiatr. Clin. N. Am.*, 14(4):877–908.

Seidel L, Walkup JT. 2006. Selective serotonin reuptake inhibitor use in the treatment of the pediatric non-obsessive-compulsive disorder anxiety disorders. *J. Child Adolesc. Psychopharmacol.*, 16(1–2):171–9.

Stahl SM. 2006. *Essential Psychopharmacology: The Prescriber's Guide*. Cambridge: Cambridge University Press.

Varley CK, Smith CJ. 2003. Anxiety disorders in the child and teen. *Pediatr. Clin. N. Am.*, 50:1107–38.

Walkup J, Labellarte M. 2001. Complications of SSRI treatment. *J. Child Adolesc. Psychopharmacol.*, 11(1):1–4.

Waslick B. 2006. Psychopharmacology interventions for pediatric anxiety disorders: a research update. *Child Adolesc. Psychiatr. Clin. N. Am.*, 15:51–71.

Whittington CJ, Kendal T, Fonagy P, Cottrell D, Cotgrove A, Boddington E. 2004. Selective serotonin reuptake inhibitors in childhood depression: systematic review of published versus unpublished data. *Lancet*, 363:1341–5.

Witek MW, Rojas V, Alonso C, Minami H, Silva RR. 2005. Review of benzodiazepine use in children and adolescents. *Psychiatr. Q.*, 76(3):283–96.

# Attention deficit/hyperactivity disorder

5

**Donald E. Greydanus, Cynthia Feucht and Eleni Tzima-Tsitsika**

## ■ Introduction

Attention-deficit/hyperactivity disorder (ADHD) is noted in 3–9% of children and adolescents, three times more commonly in males than females. The precise diagnosis depends on which diagnostic criteria the clinician uses and the reader is referred to the classification used by the *The International Classification of Diseases, 10th edn.* (ICD–10) published by the World Health Organization in 1993, the American Psychiatric Association's *Diagnostic and Statistical Manual of Mental Disorders* (DSM–IV–TR, 4th edn.), and the American Academy of Pediatrics' *The Classification of Child and Adolescent Mental Diagnoses in Primary Care: Diagnostic and Statistical Manual for Primary Care: Child and Adolescent Version* (DSM–PC).

The DSM–IV–TR presents detailed lists of symptoms and criteria for arriving at a diagnosis; the DSM–PC is used in the USA in primary care offices and is based on the DSM–IV–TR. The ICD–10 is typically used by insurance companies, provides flexibility in the diagnosis, and identifies ADHD as attention-deficit/*hyperkinetic* disorder. Other ADHD classifications may be used, depending on the training and location of the clinician in the world. The approach to ADHD in this chapter is based on the concept that ADHD is a neurobiological condition that involves the presence of *attention span dysfunction* along with variable degrees of *hyperactivity* and *impulsivity*. Table 5.1 lists criteria for good and poor outcomes in youth with ADHD.

Individuals who have problems with attention and self-control may develop considerable impairments in academic skills, social skills

**Table 5.1** Prognostic factors in ADHD.

A. *Good Prognosis*
1. High intellectual functioning
2. Strong family supports
3. Good friends
4. Accepted by their peers
5. Nurtured by their teachers

B. *Poor Prognosis*
1. Low average to borderline intellectual functioning
2. Minimal family supports
3. Few friends
4. Not accepted by their peers
5. Not nurtured by their teachers
6. Have one or more comorbid psychiatric disorders

attainment, and emotional/psychological stability. Noradrenergic and dopaminergic pathways are involved to mediate the symptoms of ADHD. If the student cannot focus sufficiently in school to learn basic information academic achievement may be impaired, complicating the ability to succeed in adult life. Table 5.2 provides a list of conditions that should be considered when a diagnosis of ADHD arises.

A careful assessment is necessary to be sure the core ADHD symptoms are not due to other mental health disorders. Also, comorbid conditions may be present and the youth can present with both ADHD and additional diagnoses (Table 5.3). Psychiatric disorders may be found in 44% of youth having ADHD; 32% have at least two psychiatric disorders, and 11% have three or more.

## ■ Evaluation

Diagnosis of ADHD is based on careful assessments of the functioning of the child or adolescent in various environments – school, home, and work (if appropriate). Information is also helpful regarding peer relations, family mental health history, family conflict history, and history of psychological trauma in the adolescent. There is no definitive test(s) for ADHD, but a comprehensive evaluation should include behavioral, psychological, and neurological testing. The assessment should look at presenting problems of the child or adolescent, differential diagnoses, and potential comorbid

**Table 5.2** Differential diagnoses of ADHD.

*Mental health disorders*

Anxiety disorders (generalized anxiety disorder, separation anxiety)

Affective (mood) disorders

Conduct disorder

Impulse-control disorders

Mental retardation

Mood disorders

Oppositional defiant disorder

Pervasive developmental disorders; autism

Psychotic disorders: schizophrenia or other dissociative disorders

Adjustment disorders

*Medical disorders*

Hyperthyroidism

Early stages of progressive neurodegenerative disorders

Subclinical epilepsy, absence seizures

Frontal lobe tumor or abscess

Fetal alcohol syndrome

Klinefelter syndrome

Angelman syndrome

Velocardiofacial syndrome

Sotos syndrome

Neurobehavioral effects of lead toxicity

Sleep disorders

Obstructive sleep apnea syndrome

Effects of chronic diseases and their drug treatments (e.g. severe asthma, migraine, cancer)

*Effects of drugs*

Drugs of abuse (e.g. phencyclidine, cocaine, CNS stimulants)

Therapeutic drugs (e.g. Phenobarbital, albuterol, corticosteroids, antihistamines)

*Effects of environment*

Child and adolescent abuse and neglect

Severely dysfunctional family dynamics

Highly gifted student in unchallenging curricular environment

Cognitively challenged student in regular classroom environment

disorders. A careful physical examination is also important along with selective laboratory tests based on findings from the medical history and examination. Records from other providers and teachers can also be very useful in the evaluation process. The patient should be screened for depression,

**Table 5.3** ADHD comorbid mental disorders.

Anxiety disorders
Mood disorders
Conduct disorder
Oppositional defiant disorder
Developmental coordination disorder
Specific learning disability
Communication disorders
Tourette disorder

**Table 5.4** Psychological management of ADHD in youth.

Psychotherapy
Cognitive-behavioral therapy (CBT)
Behavioral therapy (BT)
Psychosocial interventions:
   Support groups
   Social skills training
   Biofeedback training
   Peer mediation to resolve interpersonal conflicts
   Family therapy
   Self-management training

anxiety disorders, and other mental health conditions. The clinician should work with appropriate consultants in psychology, psychiatry, neurology and other fields, depending on the presenting findings.

# ■ Psychological management

Various psychological treatments are available to the trained clinician to improve ADHD in the adolescent, as outlined in Table 5.4 (see Chapter 1).

There is very little research support for the efficacy of these psychological treatments except for cognitive–behavioral therapy. In the USA, most ADHD youth are treated with medication. It is our recommendation that children and youth receiving a diagnosis of ADHD should receive management involving both psychological and psychopharmacological interventions if possible. The rest of this chapter now focuses on pharmacological treatment of ADHD in youth.

# Psychopharmacologic management

There is over 60 years of research noting that medication can ameliorate ADHD symptoms in children, adolescents, and adults. Drugs used for treatment of children and adolescents with ADHD include: *stimulants, antidepressants, alpha$_2$ agonists*, and *norepinephrine reuptake inhibitors*. Principles of ADHD psychopharmacology are listed in Table 5.5.

# Stimulant drugs

Hundreds of research studies on patients with ADHD have noted the beneficial effects of stimulant medications (Tables 5.6 and 5.7). Approximately 75% or more of those with ADHD note some benefit, and the use of medication has become a standard part of management for these patients by many clinicians. The most comprehensive study today was arranged by the National Institute of Mental Health (NIMH) in the USA; this research was named the NIMH Collaborative Multisite Multimodal Treatment Study of Children with Attention Deficit/Hyperactivity Disorder, Combined type (or the *MTA* study). It involved 579 children aged 7–9.9 years of age and documented the efficacy of methylphenidate (MPH) for these children above that of psychological therapies; the second best management strategy was the combination of MPH plus cognitive–behavioral therapy.

## Methylphenidate preparations

Methylphenidate is the stimulant most commonly prescribed for patients with ADHD since its production starting in 1957. Methylphenidate is as a nonamphetamine sympathomimetic agent, with mild CNS stimulant properties. Its putative mechanism of action is through activation of brain stem and cortical arousal systems. Its beneficial effect on attention span dysfunction is based on selective binding of the presynaptic dopamine transporter in the CNS striatal and prefrontal areas, leading to rise in extracellular dopamine. It also causes a blockade of the CNS norepinephrine transporter in the norepinephrine system. Beneficial effects of stimulant medication may include enhanced concentration, reduced hyperarousal, reduced impulsivity, reduced motor restlessness (i.e. less gross/fine motor movement), and less aggressive and/or antisocial behavior. There is no

**Table 5.5** Principles of psychopharmacologic management for ADHD.

1. Educate the patient and parents ("family") about the purpose of these medications; clarify the goals of medications (improving concentration, decreasing impulsivity, others). The clinician should avoid focusing only on medication in the clinical encounter, which implies to families that medication use alone should be the remedy to all problems. It further implies that when things are not going well, the problem must be with the choice or dose of medication. This shifts responsibility for problems completely to the clinician who must then urgently find the right medication.
2. Be sure the patient and parents understand that medications are not curative.
3. Correct any "myths" about medication the family may have. For example, medication will not correct family problems (i.e. alcoholism in a parent, contentious custody battles).
4. Wait for the patient/family to approve of a trial medication period before embarking on medication management. Do not force medication on a child or adolescent.
5. Educate the patient/family about potential side effects of medications and how you will deal with them; follow these patients on a regular basis to monitor efficacy and adverse effects.
6. Provide a thorough evaluation of the patient and family to determine possible comorbidities that may benefit from other medications.
7. Be supportive of other management tools (i.e. psychoeducation strategies, behavioral therapy).
8. Begin with a low dose and increase slowly until identified target symptoms are sufficiently improved; stop the medication(s) if side effects are unacceptable or upper medication levels are reached without amelioration of target symptoms.
9. Specific medications and doses may vary from patient to patient and are identified by careful trial and error. Medication(s) that are helpful may change as the child emerges to adolescence and adulthood.
10. Adolescents may require a medication dose higher than needed for adults because of increased renal clearance of drugs, lower body fat percentage, increased liver metabolism, or idiosyncratic medication metabolism.
11. Strive to achieve complete syndrome remission if feasible (rather than settling for symptom improvement).
12. Share responsibility explicitly by clearly stating what issues the family must work on, the school must work on, the child or adolescent must work on, and the physician must work on.

*Source:* Modified with permission from Greydanus DE *et al.* 2003. Attention-deficit/hyperactivity disorder in children and adolescents: Interventions for a complex costly clinical conundrum. *Pediatr Clin N. Am*, 50:1061–2.

**Table 5.6** Methylphenidate preparations.

| Brand name | Dosage form | Dosing regimen | | Maximum per day | Duration of effect in hours |
|---|---|---|---|---|---|
| | | Start | Titrate weekly | | |
| *Active ingredient: d,l,methylphenidate* | | | | | |
| Ritalin; Generic form available | Scored tablets: 5, 10, 20 mg | 5 mg 2–3 times/day; 1 dose before breakfast, 1 before lunch | 5–10 mg; Give a third dose in the afternoon if needed | Not to exceed 20 mg/dose; 60 mg/day | 3–4 |
| Methylin | Scored tablets: 5, 10, 20 mg; chewable tablets: 2.5, 5, 10 mg; oral solution: 5 mg/ml, 10 mg/ml | 5 mg 2–3 times/day; 1 dose before breakfast, 1 before lunch | 5–10 mg; Give a third dose in the afternoon if needed | Not to exceed 20 mg/dose; 60 mg/day | 4–8 |
| Ritalin SR | Sustained release tablets: 20 mg | 20 mg before breakfast | 20 mg; Give a second dose in afternoon if needed; for desired dose and duration, short-acting form may be used | 60 mg | 6–8 |
| Metadate ER | Extended release tablets: 10, 20 mg | 10 mg before breakfast | 10 mg; Give a second dose in afternoon if needed | 60 mg | 4–8 |
| Methylin ER | Extended release tablets: 10, 20 mg | 10 mg before breakfast | 10 mg; Give a second dose in afternoon if needed | 60 mg | 4–8 |

*(cont.)*

**Table 5.6** (*cont.*)

| Brand name | Dosage form | Dosing regimen | | Maximum per day | Duration of effect in hours |
| | | Start | Titrate weekly | | |
| --- | --- | --- | --- | --- | --- |
| Metadate CD | Extended release capsules: 10, 20, 30 mg. Can be sprinkled | 20 mg before breakfast | 20 mg; Give a second dose in the afternoon if needed | 60 mg | 4–8 |
| Ritalin LA | Long acting capsules: 10, 20, 30, 40 mg; can be sprinkled | 10 mg before breakfast | 5–10 mg; Use short-acting form (Ritalin) to titrate if needed | 60 mg | 4–8 |
| Concerta | Capsules: 18, 27, 36, 54 mg; do not split or chew or crush | 18 mg before breakfast | 18 mg | 72 mg | 8–12 |
| Daytrana | Transdermal patch: 10, 15, 20, 30 mg | 10 mg patch applied 2 hours before desired effect; remove 9 hours later | 10 mg | 30 mg | 12 |
| *Active ingredient: d, methylphenidate* | | | | | |
| Focalin | Scored tablets: 2.5, 5, 10 mg | 2.5 mg 1 to 2 times a day | 2.5 mg; Give a third dose in afternoon if needed. | 30 mg | 4–5 |
| Focalin XR | Extended release capsules: 5, 10 mg; can be sprinkled | 5 mg before breakfast | 5 mg; Give a second dose in afternoon if needed; for desired dose and duration short acting form (Focalin) may be used | 30 mg | 8–12 |

**Table 5.7** Amphetamine preparations.

| Brand name | Dosage form | Dosing regimen | | Maximum per day | Duration of effect in hours |
| | | Start | Titrate weekly | | |
|---|---|---|---|---|---|
| *Active Ingredient: Dextroamphetamine* | | | | | |
| Dexedrine Generic form available | Tablets: 5 mg | 5 mg 1 to 2 times/day | 5 mg | 40 mg | 4–6 |
| Dextrostat Generic form | Scored tablets: 5, 10 mg | 2.5–5 mg 1 to 2 times/day | 5 mg | 40 mg | 4–6 |
| | Extended release capsules: 5, 10, 20 mg | 5 mg 1 to 2 times/day | 5 mg | 40 mg | 4–6 |
| Dexedrine Spansule | Spansules: 5, 10, 15 mg; can be sprinkled | 5 mg before breakfast | 5 mg | 45 mg | 6–10 |
| *Active Ingredient: Mixed salts of amphetamine (dextroamphetamine plus levoamphetamine)* | | | | | |
| Adderall Generic form available | Tablets: 5, 7.5, 10, 12.5, 15, 20, 30 mg | 5–10 mg 1 to 2 times per day; 1 dose before breakfast, second before lunch | 5–10 mg | 40 mg | 4–6 |
| Adderall XR | Extended release capsules: 5, 10, 15, 20, 25, 30 mg; can be sprinkled | 5–10 mg before breakfast | 5–10 mg | 30 mg | 8–12 |

**Table 5.8** Reasons for failure of methylphenidate (MPH).

- Inaccurate diagnosis
- Comorbid disorders that overshadow the ADHD
- Medication doses that are too high or not high enough
- Medication is diverted to others in or outside the family
- Intolerable medication side effects
- Medication is used as a drug of abuse for its euphoric effects
- Patient and/or family not accepting of medication
- Patient does not respond to MPH but does to other stimulants or alternative medications
- Patient does not respond to medications of any kind

*Source:* Modified with permission from Greydanus DE *et al.* 2002. Psychopharmacology of ADHD in adolescents. *Adolesc. Med.*, 13:604.

correlation between weight of the patient and optimal MPH dose, and plasma levels of MPH are not useful. A number of tools are used to assess effectiveness, such as patient/family interviews, parent ratings, school grades or reports, and others. Reasons for failure of MPH to be effective are listed in Table 5.8.

Various immediate-release or short-acting preparations of MPH have been popular until recently, when a number of longer-acting MPH products were developed. Pharmaceutical companies have developed a variety of alternative MPH preparations over the past decade and they are listed in Table 5.6.

There are no unbiased studies available at this time to tell the clinician and patient which of these products are superior, and the clinicians and patients must simply find out by a process of "trial and error" which product is best for the individual patient. If a patient has difficulty swallowing pills, some of the longer-acting products can be opened and sprinkled on apple sauce.

## Amphetamine preparations

The beneficial effects of amphetamine on ADHD date back to 1937. The amphetamines are noncatecholamine, sympathomimetic amines that act as CNS stimulants. Their putative mechanism of action involves reuptake blockade of neurotransmitters (dopamine and norepinephrine) into presynaptic neurons, as well as an increased release of those neurotransmitters

**Table 5.9** Potential side effects of stimulant drugs.

Headache*
Nausea/vomiting*
Anorexia*
Insomnia (delayed onset of sleep)

Weight loss*
Moodiness (irritability)

Tachycardia
Palpitations
Sudden cardiac death
Increase in blood pressure
"Unmasking" of Tourette syndrome
Rebound phenomenon

Reduced seizure threshold
Irritability/ restlessness
Emotional lability
Appearance of psychosis or psychotic features

Growth retardation (at higher doses, over longer times, in those with short stature
   or slow axial growth)
Skin rash (rare)

*Commonly seen side effects
*Source:* Modified with permission from Greydanus DE *et al.* 2002.
Psychopharmacology of ADHD in adolescents. *Adolesc. Med.*, 13:607.

into the synaptic cleft. Amphetamines are available as dextroamphetamine sulfate (the dextro isomer of *d,l* amphetamine sulfate) or as mixed amphetamine salts (dextroamphetamine plus levoamphetamine). The potential adverse effects of amphetamines are the same as MPH (Table 5.9). Amphetamine products that are available are listed in Table 5.7.

## Pemoline

In 1996, the USFDA (Washington, DC) gave its first black box warning for pemoline due to rare irreversible liver failure that may occur and denoting its place in ADHD therapy as third line versus first line. In June 1999, an additional black box warning was issued describing 21 cases of hepatic failure including 13 deaths or liver transplants since marketing. In October 2005, the FDA reviewed the overall risk profile and deemed the benefits did not outweigh the risks associated with its use. Pemoline was withdrawn from the market in 2005 and is no longer available for use in the USA, UK, Canada, and other countries.

## Contraindications for stimulant use

Unless stated otherwise, it is assumed that any medication will have as a contraindication sensitivity to that medication or any of its ingredients. Patients with significant levels of anxiety, inner tension, or psychomotor agitation should not be on psychostimulants. Other contraindications to stimulants include drug and alcohol dependence, glaucoma, psychosis, and hyperthyroidism. Due to potential cardiovascular side effects, stimulants should not be used in patients with uncontrolled hypertension, symptomatic cardiovascular disorder (i.e. angina, heart failure), serious structural cardiac abnormalities, cardiomyopathy, and serious heart rhythm abnormalities. The use of stimulants in the presence of motor tic disorder or Tourette's syndrome is relatively contraindicated along with a history of epilepsy. Stimulants should not be combined with monoamine oxidase inhibitors since this combination can lead to a hypertensive crisis. Therefore 2 weeks should be allowed between prescribing a stimulant and discontinuing a monoamine oxidase inhibitor. Mixing a stimulant with a tricyclic antidepressant may lead to sudden death from cardiac arrhythmias in rare cases. Methylphenidate can interfere with the metabolism of some anticonvulsant drugs, such as phenytoin and phenobarbital. Agents that inhibit cytochrome P450 2D6 isoenzyme (i.e. paroxetine and quinidine) may increase the effects of methylphenidate.

Methylphenidate appears to be safe to use in children with developmental disabilities with ADHD and a seizure disorder (see Chapter 10). The seizure disorder should be well-controlled and contraindicated conditions (i.e. psychosis) should be excluded before MPH is started.

## Side effects of stimulants

Side effects of stimulants are listed in Table 5.9, some of which are transient, and can be reduced if the patient starts with a low dose and slowly increases the dosage to maximize benefit with reduced side effects.

Nausea or emesis that may occur with stimulants often improves if the medication is taken with meals. Dizziness occurs in some patients and is worse with short-acting stimulants versus long-acting types (see Tables 5.6 and 5.7). If dizziness occurs, look for dehydration or blood pressure changes and treat as necessary. Headaches may develop while taking stimulants and this may be related to peak plasma levels or related to drug withdrawal. A change to a different formulation may provide symptomatic relief. There is no indication that the use of stimulant medication increases the risk of substance abuse.

The phenomenon of delayed growth in children or growing adolescents on stimulants remains controversial and seems to be, in part, related to appetite suppression with decreased caloric intake. It appears to be a transient effect, and most children eventually seem to attain expected adult height. Youth on stimulants who are not growing properly need careful supervision. If the appetite is blunted while on stimulants, a number of measures can be taken, including taking food when the stimulant wears off (as in the evening), using high-caloric foods or nutritional supplements, taking the patient off stimulants when not in school (such as during vacation or on weekends), and trying other anti-ADHD medications.

*Tolerance* may develop in some youth receiving high stimulant doses and chronic abuse. Management involves tapering off the stimulant and trying a different anti-ADHD medication. Rebound can develop in which increased ADHD symptoms (i.e. irritability, sadness, and excitability) develop as the stimulant effect wears off. This can be managed by giving a smaller immediate-release dose in the afternoon or changing to a sustained release product. Stimulants may interfere with sleep and this side effect tends to diminish with time. In addition to stimulant side effect, the child with sleep disturbances should be carefully evaluated for other causes of sleep disturbances. Administering the last dose of the day earlier, eliminating or reducing the last dose of the day, or the use of a long-acting preparation are some of the strategies that may help with sleep problems. Pharmacological options for sleep problems in children are limited. Although drugs such as tricyclic antidepressants, alpha$_2$ agonists (i.e. clonidine), trazodone, or melatonin have been used, potential complications of combination of these drugs with stimulants must be carefully considered.

Attention deficit/hyperactivity disorder is found in 50–75% of patients with Tourette Syndrome (TS) and TS may become apparent in some children or adolescents after starting stimulant drugs. Research does not suggest that stimulant medications cause TS and the presence of tics is a relative, not absolute contraindication to stimulant medication. Youth with both ADHD and TS may be given both stimulant medications (if effective) and anti-tic medication (such as risperidone, haloperidol, or pimozide). If the tics are worsened by the stimulant drugs, other anti-ADHD medications may be tried that do not typically worsen tics such as alpha$_2$ agonists (i.e. clonidine or guanfacine) or atomoxetine. Bupropion may improve ADHD but worsens tics and should be avoided.

## Cardiovascular side effects

Because of reports of serious cardiovascular adverse events in recent years the USFDA has required that a strong warning should be placed on the label of stimulant drugs (See Box 3.1, Chapter 3). Before starting a child or adolescent on a stimulant drug a careful cardiovascular screening is recommended with the goal of identifying the child or adolescent at risk for serious underlying cardiovascular disease and adverse events related to stimulant use. Key elements to be included in cardiovascular screening are listed in Table 5.10.

### How to monitor patients on stimulants

In cases of long-term use of stimulants, periodic complete blood count, with differential and platelet count, are recommended. Height and weight should be monitored routinely, and any significant slowing should prompt further evaluation and possible discontinuation of the stimulant medication. Blood pressure and pulse should be checked at each medication visit, as both values can increase with stimulant treatment.

## ■ Nonstimulant medications

### Atomoxetine

Atomoxetine is a nonstimulant medication that is a selective inhibitor of norepinephrine reuptake. Its actions include the blockade of the presynaptic norepinephrine and dopamine transporter in the prefrontal cortex. In addition to methylphenidate, amphetamines and atomoxetine are the only medications currently approved by the USFDA for use in children with ADHD. Atomoxetine can be used in those not wishing to take a stimulant, where stimulant or other medications are ineffective or in patients with anxiety symptoms. Atomoxetine is available as a capsule for oral administration in the 10, 18, 25, 40, 60, 80, and 100 mg dosage forms. For the child or adolescent weighing 70 kg or less the recommended starting dose is

**Table 5.10** Cardiovascular screening.

*Personal history*
Exertional chest pain
Shortness of breath
Presyncope
Syncope
Dizziness
Palpitations
Fatigue
Recent febrile illness
Congenital heart disease
Heart murmur
Hypertension
Lipid disorder or abnormalities

*Past history*
Kawasaki's disease
Rheumatic fever

*Family history*
Marfan syndrome
Cardiomyopathy
Long QT syndrome
Premature cardiac death (before age 50)
Hypertension
Lipid disorders

*Cardiovascular exam*
Heart rate; Blood pressure; Delayed femoral arterial pulses (coarctation of aorta)
Systolic ejection murmur that intensifies with standing or Valsalva maneuver and
   diminishes with squatting (hypertrophic cardiomyopathy)
Decrescendo diastolic murmur of aortic valve insufficiency (may be present in
   Marfan syndrome)
Holosystolic murmur of mitral valve insufficiency (may be present in Marfan
   syndrome)
Systolic ejection murmur or midsystolic clicks (mitral valve prolapse)

0.5 mg/kg/day that is increased at least every 3 days to 1.2 mg/kg/day given
as a single dose or in 2 divided doses. The maximum dose should not exceed
1.4 mg/kg/day or 100 mg per day. For patients who weigh more than 70 kg
the recommended starting dose is 40 mg per day that can be increased up
to 80 mg per day given as a single or 2 divided doses, not to exceed 100 mg
per day. The duration of atomoxetine effect is 18–24 hours.

**Table 5.11** Atomoxetine side effects.

Anorexia
Constipation
Dry mouth
Nausea
Emesis
Sedation
Fatigue
Headache
Dizziness
Mood swings
Suicidal ideations
Aggressive behavior
Dyspepsia
Stomachache
Growth delay
Tachycardia
Hepatotoxicity

Table 5.11 lists potential adverse effects of atomoxetine. Atomoxetine has been associated with an increased risk of mydriasis, and should not be used in patients with narrow angle glaucoma. Due to reporting of several cases of severe liver injury, the manufacturer's package insert was modified in December 2004 to recommend baseline liver function tests with periodic monitoring. Children and adolescents should be monitored for an increased risk of suicidality due to reports of increased risk of suicidal ideation and behavior, and atomoxetine carries the US FDA black box warning similar to that for antidepressants (see Box 3.2, Chapter 3). It also carries a similar warning for potential hepatotoxicity. Patients on atomoxetine should also be monitored for suicidality in a manner similar to that recommended for children and adolescents on antidepressants (see Appendix 3.1, Chapter 3 and see Chapter 6). There is no increase in drug addiction, drug diversion, cardiovascular complications, or tics. Drug–drug interactions can occur with inhibitors of the cytochrome P450, 2D6 isoenzyme, including selective serotonin reuptake inhibitors.

## Tricyclic antidepressants

Research studies note that tricyclic antidepressants (TCAs) may be useful in some patients with ADHD, and are considered an alternative to stimulant

**Table 5.12** Indications for tricyclic antidepressants.

ADHD (Attention deficit/hyperactivity disorder)
Aggression disorders
Anxiety disorders (as panic disorder or obsessive-compulsive disorder)
Depression
Enuresis
Insomnia
Migraine prophylaxis
Tourette syndrome
Neuropathy

medications if stimulants are not beneficial or are contraindicated. Antidepressants may be a superior choice in those patients with prominent anxiety symptoms or addictive personalities. Table 5.12 lists other indications for the use of TCAs. Tricyclic antidepressants that have been used for the treatment of ADHD in children and adolescents include imipramine (2–5 mg/kg/day or 50–200 mg/day), amitriptyline (1–1.5 mg/kg/day or 50–200 mg/day), and nortriptyline (1–3 mg/kg/day or 20–100 mg/day). The TCAs block reuptake, to varying degrees, of the monoamine neurotransmitters (norepinephrine and serotonin) into the presynaptic neurons. They also have significant anticholinergic and antihistaminic effects.

## Tricyclic antidepressant monitoring

Tricyclic antidepressants should be initiated with a low dose at bedtime and titrated slowly with careful monitoring. A baseline electrocardiogram (ECG) should be obtained and repeated with each dose titration. The ECG should be evaluated for any development of cardiac arrhythmias. The PR interval, QRS interval and $QT_c$ should be measured to detect cardiac side effects. Upper limits of acceptable parameters are: PR interval not to exceed 0.21 seconds, QRS not to exceed over 30% of its base (not over 120 milliseconds) and the $QT_c$ not to exceed over 0.460 second. Serum TCA levels are important to maintain medication levels within a therapeutic range (Table 6.4, Chapter 6), though increasing efficacy is not necessarily correlated with increasing serum levels and toxicity may occur even in a "safe" or therapeutic range. A serum prolactin should be performed if the patient develops gynecomastia or menstrual irregularities. Similar to other antidepressant class of drugs, TCAs carry the US FDA black box warning for

**Table 5.13** Tricyclic antidepressant side effects.

Blurred vision
Confusion
Constipation
Nausea/vomiting
Dizziness
Drowsiness and sedation

Dry mouth
ECG changes
Cardiac arrhythmias
Syndrome of inappropriate antidiuretic hormone secretion
Orthostatic hypotension
Decrease in seizure threshold

Skin rash
Sudden death
Tachycardia
Tremor
Restlessness
Urinary retention
Weight gain
Suicidal ideations
Sexual dysfunction

*Source:* Modified with permission from Greydanus DE *et al.*
Attention-deficit/hyperactivity disorder in children and
adolescents: interventions for a complex costly clinical
conundrum. *Pediatr. Clin. N. Am.*, 50:1079, 2003.

suicidality in children and adolescents and recommended clinical monitoring guidelines should be followed for patients on TCAs (see Chapters 3
and 6).

Table 5.13 lists adverse effects of TCAs. Tricyclic antidepressants tend to
cause less rebound effect than stimulants. Sedation can be severe and is
worse with imipramine than with amitriptyline or nortriptyline. Tricyclic
antidepressant-induced tremor can be alleviated by careful reduction in
TCA dose or adding propranolol (10–40 mg per day). If agitation develops as a result of the TCA, lowering of the dose may provide benefit or
changing to an alternative medication may become necessary. Mania may
develop if a TCA is added to someone with latent bipolar disorder and psychosis may develop if a TCA is added to someone with latent schizophrenia.

Nausea, emesis, fatigue, or worsening behavior may develop if the TCA is stopped abruptly resulting in a discontinuation syndrome. Tricyclic antidepressants may reduce the seizure threshold and should be used with caution in patients with a history of a seizure disorder. With the exception of bupropion and mirtazapine, all of the commonly used antidepressants can cause hyponatremia and/or syndrome of inappropriate secretion of antidiuretic hormone (SIADH).

Tricyclic antidepressants are metabolized by the cytochrome P450 system and care must be taken when adding other medications to TCAs. For example, toxic TCA levels may occur when combining TCAs with SSRIs. The combination of MPH and a TCA may lead to rising TCA levels as well. The TCAs should not be used concomitantly with MAOIs or with medications that prolong the $QT_c$ interval. They should be used with caution in patients with a history of seizures, narrow-angle glaucoma, cardiovascular disease, anorexia, hyperthyroidism, or patients receiving thyroid supplementation. Respiratory depression and death may develop after combining alcohol and TCAs.

## Alpha₂ agonists

### Clonidine

Clonidine is a presynaptic, central-acting alpha₂-adrenergic agonist that is used by some clinicians to manage ADHD symptoms, though it may take 4–6 weeks to achieve full benefit and is less effective than stimulants. These agents stimulate brainstem alpha₂-adrenoreceptors, effectively reducing CNS sympathetic outflow. Clonidine is used as an alternative or adjunctive medication to MPH. It is often given with MPH to treat the insomnia related to MPH. Clonidine is also used to manage Tourette's syndrome, posttraumatic stress disorder, and severe aggressiveness with conduct disorder or oppositional defiant disorder (see Chapters 7, 10, and 12).

Table 5.14 lists potential adverse effects of clonidine. Clonidine is available in the form of 0.1 mg, 0.2 mg, and 0.3 mg tablets and transdermal patch. The dosage of clonidine generally ranges from 0.05 mg to 0.3 mg daily (maximum 0.4 mg/day) taken orally given in 2–3 divided doses or with most of the medication administered at nighttime. A gradual titration when initiating clonidine and tapering when discontinuing is recommended. Abrupt discontinuations can result in severe rebound hypertension, cerebrovascular accidents, and sudden death.

**Table 5.14** Side effects of clonidine.

Sedation (50%)
Dry mouth
Headache
Nausea/vomiting
Constipation
Depression
Contact dermatitis (patch)
Erythema (patch)
Sexual dysfunction
Dizziness
Dysphoria
Fatigue/lethargy
Postural hypotension
Rebound phenomenon
Withdrawal effects (rebound tachycardia, severe hypertension, heart failure from
   sudden clonidine cessation)

*Source:* Modified with permission from Greydanus DE *et al.* 2002.
Psychopharmacology of ADHD in adolescents. *Adolesc. Med.*, 13:615.

Blood pressure should be monitored for hypotension and rebound hypertension. No laboratory studies are required; however, an electrocardiogram
and a thorough cardiac history should be performed prior to initiating
clonidine (see Cardiovascular screening, Table 5.10). Clonidine should not
be used in children and adolescents with structural heart disease. Iso-
lated cases of sudden death have been reported in children and adolescents taking both MPH and clonidine. The relationship between the
deaths and drug combination is unclear due to the presence of confounding
factors.

Clonidine is available as a patch which lasts 7 days. The patch may
decrease the sedation seen with the oral formulation and enhance compliance. As with any patch, dermatitis may occur at the site of the patch
application. Changing the patch site and local application of hydrocortisone usually resolves the local dermatitis. Severe dermatitis may warrant
discontinuation of clonidine. In a patient who has developed a skin reaction
switching to an oral form or changing the site of the patch application is not
recommended, as it may be associated with development of a generalized
reaction, acute urticaria, or angioedema.

**Table 5.15** Bupropion side effects.

Anorexia
Weight loss
Agitation
Nausea
Constipation
Restlessness
Dizziness
Insomnia
Headache
Tics (exacerbation)
Seizures (0.1% under 300 mg/day and 0.4% over 300 mg/day)
Suicidality

## Guanfacine

Guanfacine is an alpha$_{2A}$-adrenergic agonist related to clonidine, and also proven to benefit some children and adolescents with attention span problems of ADHD. Its use may result in fewer blood pressure problems and sedation than seen with clonidine. Adverse reactions are similar to clonidine, but there may be more agitation and headaches. Its daily dosage range is 0.5–4.0 mg.

## Bupropion

Bupropion is an antidepressant medication with noradrenergic/dopaminergic effects to improve depression and ameliorate attention dysfunction. Bupropion works by inhibiting dopamine and norepinephrine reuptake into the presynaptic neuron. Bupropion is available for oral administration as immediate release 75 mg and 100 mg tablets; 100 mg, 150 mg, and 200 mg sustained release tablets; and 150 mg and 300 mg extended release tablets. Bupropion is given in a daily dosage range of 50–300 mg (3.0–6.0 mg/kg/day) of the immediate release form; 100–150 mg twice daily as the sustained release form; and 150 mg or 300 mg once daily of the extended release form.

Table 5.15 lists side effects of bupropion. Risk for seizures (0.1% under 300 mg a day and 0.4% over 300 mg a day) is dose-dependent (>150 mg of the immediate-release formulation or >6 mg/kg/day). Buproprion should not be used in patients with a history of seizures, anorexia/bulimia, and head trauma. It should not be used concurrently with MAOIs. Bupropion carries the US FDA black box warning for suicidality risk (Box 3.2, Chapter 3) in children and adolescents and patients should be monitored for increased risk of suicidal behaviors as recommended for other antidepressant drugs (Chapters 3 and 6). Bupropion does not lead to cardiac conduction delays as seen with TCAs. Bupropion is metabolized by the cytochrome P450 system and has the potential to interact with other agents that affect the 2B6 isoenzyme (i.e. desipramine, paroxetine, sertraline, etc.).

## Venlafaxine

Venlafaxine is an atypical antidepressant (Chapter 6) that is also used by some clinicians for ADHD and is considered a second or third line agent. Venlafaxine selectively inhibits norepinephrine and serotonin reuptake and weakly inhibits dopamine uptake. Venlafaxine is available for oral administration in the form of 25, 50, 75, and 100 mg tablets. The dosage is 1–3 mg/kg/day or 37.5–225 mg per day. As with the use of other antidepressants, children and adolescents on venlafaxine should be observed for the risk of suicidality (see Chapters 3 and 6). Sustained hypertension, which is dose-related, may occur in patients receiving this antidepressant. Since mydriasis may occur, venlafaxine should not be prescribed to someone with increased intraocular pressure or at risk for acute narrow-angle glaucoma. Drug interactions with MAOIs are well-known. Venlafaxine is metabolized by numerous isoenzymes of the cytochrome P450 system and has the potential for multiple drug interactions. Caution should be exercised when adding additional medications to venlafaxine. Venlafaxine is contraindicated in individuals with heart disease.

## Modafinil

A newer agent in this category is modafinil, which acts in many ways like the sympathomimetic agents, yet is unique, in that it does not bind to catecholamine receptors nor increase adrenergic activity. Its exact mechanism of promoting alertness and wakefulness is unknown. Current FDA approved uses include narcolepsy and obstructive sleep apnea/hypopnea syndrome (OSAHS). It has not been FDA-approved for children and adolescents with ADHD. Modafinil is available for oral administration as 100 mg and

**Table 5.16** Non-research supported ADHD treatment options.

Anti-yeast medications
Chiropractic manipulation
Dietary manipulation
Electroencephalographic-biofeedback training
Herbal treatments
Megavitamin therapy
Sensory integrative training
"Herbal" products
    Acetyl carnitine
    DMAE (dimethylaminoethanol [Deaner])
    Ginkgo biloba
    Phosphatidylserine (CNS phospholipid)
    Essential fatty acids (gamma-linolenic acid, docosahexaenoic acid)

200 mg tablets. Typical dosing in children with ADHD is 50–100 mg daily. Some common side effects include headache, gastrointestinal disturbances, nervousness, dizziness, anxiety (dose-related), and insomnia. As with other stimulants, modafinil should not be used in patients with a history of cardiovascular disease or Tourette's syndrome and caution should be used in patients with a history of psychosis. Modafinil has the propensity for drug interactions since it is metabolized by the cytochrome P450 system and can act as an inducer or inhibitor of the cytochrome P450 system.

# ■ Nonmedication alternatives

Table 5.16 lists treatment options used by some clinicians but not proven to be of benefit for children, adolescents, or adults with ADHD.

# ■ Summary

Stimulants are the most effective drugs for the treatment of children and adolescents with ADHD and are the drugs of choice. The use and efficacy for stimulant drugs and atomoxetine are well established by clinical trials in children and adolescents age 6 years and above. Use of stimulant or nonstimulant drugs for the treatment of ADHD in preschool-aged children (age 5 years and younger) remains controversial and not uniformly practiced, though several studies have shown effectiveness of stimulants in children between ages 3 years and 6 years. In children and adolescents either a methylphenidate or an amphetamine preparation should be started initially. If methylphenidate proves to be ineffective, amphetamine should be tried and vice versa. This strategy has been found to be quite successful in between 80% and 90% of children and adolescents. If either stimulant is ineffective to ameliorate symptoms, there is no clear consensus as to the second line of treatment. Clinicians have used TCAs, atomoxetine, bupropion, and alpha$_2$ agonists as second line treatment in children and adolescents who do not respond to stimulant drugs with variable success. Comorbid mental disorders are common in children and adolescents with ADHD and should be appropriately treated along with the treatment of ADHD.

## SELECTED BIBLIOGRAPHY

American Academy of Pediatrics. 2000. Clinical practice guideline: diagnosis and evaluation of the child with attention-deficit/hyperactivity disorder. *Pediatrics*, 105(5):1158–70.

American Academy of Pediatrics. 2001. Clinical practice guideline: treatment of the school-aged child with attention-deficit/hyperactivity disorder. *Pediatrics*, 108(4):1033–44.

American Psychiatric Association. 2000. *Diagnostic and Statistical Manual of Mental Disorders, 4th edn., Text Revision*. Washington, DC: APA, pp. 85–93.

Arnold LE, Lindsay RL, Lopez FA *et al*. 2007. Treating ADHD with a stimulant transdermal patch. *Pediatrics*, 120:1100–6.

Atomoxetine: Strattera revisited. *Med Lett* 2004;46:65.

Barkley RA. 1998a. Attention-deficit/hyperactivity disorder. *Sci. Am.*, 279(3):66–71.

Barkley RA (Ed.). 2006. *Attention Deficit Hyperactivity Disorder: A Handbook for Diagnosis*, 3rd edn. New York: Guilford Press.

Bradley C. 1937. The behavior of children receiving benzedrine. *Am. J. Psychiatry*, 94:577–85.

Clarke SD. 2000. ADHD in adolescence. *J. Adolesc. Health*, l27:77–8.

Dreyer BP. 2006. The diagnosis and management of ADHD in preschool children: The state of our knowledge and practice. *Curr. Probl. Pediatr. Adolesc. Health Care*, 36:6–30.

Gilchrist RH, Arnold LE. 2008. Long-term efficacy of ADHD pharmacotherapy in children. *Pediatr. Ann.*, 37:46–51.

Greydanus DE, Sloane MA, Rappley MD. 2002. Psychopharmacology of ADHD in adolescents. *Adolesc. Med.*, 13:599–624.

Greydanus DE. 2003. Psychopharmacology of ADHD in adolescents: Quo vadis? *Psychiatr. Times*, 20:5–9.

Greydanus DE, Pratt HD, Sloane MA *et al*. 2003. Attention-deficit/hyperactivity disorder in children and adolescents: interventions for a complex costly clinical conundrum. *Pediatr. Clin. N. Am.*, 50:1049–92.

Greydanus DE, Patel DR. 2005. The adolescent and substance abuse: Current concepts. *Curr. Probl. Pediatr. Adolesc. Health Care*, 35(3):78–98.

Greydanus DE, Pratt HD. 2006. Attention deficit hyperactivity disorder. In *Behavioral Pediatrics, 2nd edn.*, New York: iUniverse, pp. 107–42.

Greydanus DE, Pratt HD, Patel DR. 2007. Attention deficit hyperactivity disorder across the lifespan. *Disease-a-Month*, 53(2):65–132.

Jensen PS, Hinshaw SP, Swanson JM *et al.* 2001. Findings from the NIMH Multimodal Treatment Study of ADHD (MTA): Implications and applications for primary care providers. *J. Dev. Behav. Pediatr.*, 22:60–73.

Lerner M, Wigan T. 2008. Long-term safety of stimulant medications used to treat children with ADHD. *Pediatr. Ann.*, 37:37–45.

Lopez FA. 2006. ADHD: New pharmacologic treatments on the horizon. *Develop. Behav. Pediatrics*, 27(5):410–16.

National Institute of Mental Health. 2000. NIMH Research on Treatment for Attention Deficit Hyperactivity Disorder (ADHD): The Multimodal Treatment Study – Questions and Answers. Available at http://www.nimh.nih.gov/events/mtaqa.cfm.

National Institute of Mental Health (NIMH). 2001. Attention Deficit Hyperactivity Disorder. NIH Publication No. 01–4589. Available at http://www.nimh.nih.gov/publicat/helpchild.cfm.

Pliszka SR, Greenhill LL, Crismon ML *et al.* 2001. The Texas children's medication algorithm project: report of the Texas consensus conference panel on medication treatment of childhood. attention-deficit/hyperactivity disorder. Part I. *J. Am. Acad. Child. Adolesc. Psychiatry*, 39:900–19.

Pliszka SR, Crismon ML, Hughes CW *et al.* 2006. The Texas Children's Medication Algorithm Project: revision of the algorithm for pharmacology of attention-deficit/hyperactivity disorder. *J. Am. Acad. Child Adolesc. Psychiatry*, 45(6):642–57.

Rappley MD. 2005. ADHD. *N. Engl. J. Med.*, 352:123–5.

Reiff MI, Stein MT. 2003. ADHD evaluation and diagnosis: a practical approach to office practice. *Pediatr. Clin. N. Am.*, 50:1019–48.

Schubiner H, Robin AL, Young J. 2003. Attention-deficit/hyperactivity disorder in adolescent males. *Adolesc. Med.*, 14:663–76.

Solanto MV, Arnsten AFT, Castellanos FX. 2001. The neuroscience of stimulant drug action in ADHD. In Solanto MV, Arnsten AFT, Castellanos FX (Eds.) *Stimulant Drugs and ADHD*. London: Oxford University Press, pp. 355–79.

Stahl SM. 2006. *Essential Psychopharmacology: The Prescriber's Guide*. Cambridge: Cambridge University Press.

Staufer WB, Greydanus DE. 2005. Attention-deficit/hyperactivity disorder psychopharmacology for college students. *Pediatr. Clin. N. Am.*, 52:71–84.

Swanson JM, MTA Cooperative Group. 2004. National Institute of Mental Health Multimodal Treatment Study of ADHD Follow-up: changes in effectiveness and growth after the end of treatment. *Pediatrics*, 113:762–9.

Tallian K. 2006. Pharmacotherapy of ADHD. In Schumock G, Brundage D, Chapman M *et al.* (Eds.) *Pharmacotherapy Self-Assessment Program, 5th edn. Chronic*

*Illnesses IV and Pediatrics*. Kansas City, MO: American College of Clinical Pharmacy, pp. 275–96.

Thomson Healthcare, Inc. 2007. *Physicians' Desk Reference, 61st edn*. Montvale, NJ: Thomson Healthcare Inc.

Van Cleave J, Leslie LK. 2008. Approaching ADHD as a chronic condition: implications for Long-term adherence. *Pediatr. ANN.*, 37:19–26.

Varley C. 2000. Sudden death of a child treated with imipramine. *J. Child Adolesc. Psychopharmacol.*, 10:321–5.

Varley CK. 2001. Sudden death related to selected tricyclic antidepressants in children: epidemiology, mechanisms and clinical implications. *Paediatr. Drugs*, 3:613–27.

Wender EH. 2002. Managing stimulant medication for attention-deficit/hyperactivity disorder: an update. *Pediatr. Rev.*, 23:234–6.

Wolraich ML, Felice ME. 1986. *The Classification of Child and Adolescent Mental Diagnoses in Primary Care: Diagnostic and Statistical Manual for Primary Care (DSM-PC): Child and Adolescent Version*. Elk Grove Village, IL: American Academy of Pediatrics, pp. 93–110.

Wolraich ML, Wibbelsman CJ, Brown TE. 2005. ADHD: a review. *Pediatrics*, 115:749–57.

Zito JM, Safer DJ, dosReis S *et al.* 2003. Psychotropic practice patterns for youth. A 10-year perspective. *Arch. Pediatr. Adolesc. Med.*, 157:17–25.

# Child and adolescent depression

## 6

Sadness is one of the basic human emotions, and is usually associated with a current or past tragic event, such as the loss of a loved one. Depression is a more sustained state of sadness (or anger – see below) which can either arise spontaneously or follow disruptive events in the person's life. Untreated, depression can lead to morbidity and mortality, and is a significant risk factor for suicide.

The goal of this chapter is to guide the primary care clinician in the proper selection and management of medications for the treatment of depression in children and adolescents.

## ■ Definition

The clinical syndrome of major depressive disorder (MDD) is diagnosed in younger people using the same criteria as those used for adults, with some modifications made for developmental differences. For example, the 2-weeks of near-constant depressed mood can be experienced as irritability or angry mood (rather than sadness) in children and adolescents. Instead of weight loss, children may fail to gain weight appropriately. A particularly meaningful symptom is anhedonia, or the loss of pleasure in usually enjoyable activities; this seems to be fairly specific for depression in younger people. A useful mnemonic to help document the signs and symptoms of MDD is *SIGECAPS* (Table 6.1).

There are other diagnoses to consider when evaluating a depressed child or adolescent, and those will be described in the section on Differential diagnosis below.

**Table 6.1** Criteria (SIGECAPS) for the diagnosis of MDD.

Two weeks of sad/irritable mood[a] and at least four of the following:
Sleep disturbance, either insomnia or hypersomnia
Interest in activities is diminished or absent[a]
Guilt, or other thoughts of self-blame or low self-worth
Energy is low and the person fatigues easily
Concentration is poor, thinking and decision-making impaired[a]
Appetite is poor and/or weight is lost (or not gained appropriately)
Psychomotor retardation or agitation[b]
Suicidal thoughts, plans, or attempts

[a] Self-reported or observed by others
[b] Must be observed by others

# ■ Epidemiology

At any given time before puberty, 1–2% of children will experience a depressive disorder. During, or after, puberty the prevalence of depression increases to 3–8% of adolescents. Considering all of childhood, by the end of adolescence about 1 out of 5 individuals will have had a diagnosable depressive disorder.

# ■ Differential diagnosis/comorbidity

There are several clinical conditions in which depressed mood is the focal symptom (Table 6.2). The DSM–IV–TR requires that the first level of the diagnostic process eliminate medical disorders and the effects of harmful substances as possible causes of the depression. The next level of evaluation attempts to identify symptom clusters that can be categorized into specific diagnoses, such as MDD, dysthymic disorder, bipolar disorder (depressed episode), or adjustment disorder with depressed mood. For depression that does not meet any specific criteria, but is significant enough to cause distress or impair functioning, the diagnosis of depressive disorder not otherwise specified (NOS) can be used.

Depression in younger people is highly comorbid with anxiety disorders, which tends to be the separation anxiety type in children, and social anxiety type in adolescents. Anxiety often precedes the depression in younger children. Depression is also comorbid with – and is commonly preceded by – attention deficit/hyperactivity disorder (ADHD), oppositional defiant

**Table 6.2** Differential diagnosis of depression.

Mood disorder[a] due to a general medical condition
Substance induced mood disorder[a]
Major depressive disorder
Dysthymic disorder
Bipolar disorder, most recent (current) episode depressed
Adjustment disorder with depressed mood
Depressive disorder not otherwise specified

[a] Either with depressive features or with major depressive-like episode.

disorder (ODD), and conduct disorder (CD) (especially in adolescents). Depression also predisposes to the use of substances (including nicotine) in adolescents, especially if CD is also present.

# Psychopharmacology

The decision to initiate pharmacotherapy to treat MDD in a child or adolescent is predicated on two main factors: (1) in mild to moderate depression, the patient has failed to respond to an adequate trial (4–6 weeks) of psychosocial treatment; (2) the patient is experiencing a more severe depression, with marked dysfunction, agitation, hopelessness, suicidal risk, and/or psychosis.

## Medication classification and mechanism of action

The actual pathophysiology of depression is unknown, but is most commonly attributed to a disruption of the catecholamine circuits in the limbic system. The antidepressant medications modify catecholamine levels, with the ultimate effects of down-regulation of post-synaptic receptors, changes in second-messenger processes, and normalization of mood. Mood stabilizers – lithium and some anticonvulsants – are sometimes used to augment the effects of antidepressants when treating MDD. They are also used to treat the depressive phase of bipolar disorder. Antipsychotic medications are used to treat the psychotic symptoms associated with severe depression. In some treatment protocols they are also used to treat bipolar depression.

The classes of medications used in the treatment of depressive disorders, and their putative modes of action, are listed below.

(1) Selective serotonin reuptake inhibitors (SSRIs). These medications block the reuptake of serotonin into presynaptic neurons.

(2) Other (newer) classes. Nefazodone works via antagonism at the postsynaptic serotonin 5-HT$_2$ receptor; it also blocks presynaptic serotonin reuptake. Mirtazapine is an antagonist of the presynaptic norepinephrine $\alpha_2$ receptor; it also blocks postsynaptic 5-HT$_2$ and 5-HT$_3$ receptors. Venlafaxine and duloxetine are selective serotonin/norepinephrine reuptake inhibitors. Bupropion works by inhibiting dopamine and norepinephrine reuptake into the presynaptic neuron.

(3) Tricyclic antidepressants. The tricyclic antidepressants (TCAs) block reuptake – to varying degrees – of the monoamine neurotransmitters (dopamine, norepinephrine, serotonin) into the presynaptic neurons. They also have significant anticholinergic and antihistaminic effects.

(4) Monoamine oxidase inhibitors (MAOIs). These medications prevent the breakdown of the monoamine neurotransmitters present in the terminal portion of presynaptic neurons.

(5) Mood stabilizers. Lithium affects neuronal sodium transport, and may affect neuronal processing of the catecholamines. Proposed theories of how the anticonvulsants work include neuronal membrane stabilization, the inhibition of excitatory amino acids, and/or the elevation of inhibitory neurotransmitters.

(6) Antipsychotics. The exact mechanisms by which the newer antipsychotic agents stabilize mood are unknown.

## Dosages

The dosing of antidepressants in children and adolescents is based on data from a few studies in those age groups, extrapolations from adult studies, and mostly anecdotal clinical experience. Dosages in Table 6.3 are listed as a daily milligram range and/or daily milligram-per-kilogram range for each medication.

## Side effects (adverse effects)

Since 2004, the US FDA has required that the prescribing information for all available antidepressants carry a "black box" (i.e. serious) warning regarding the increase in suicidal ideation and behavior associated with

**Table 6.3** Medications used for the treatment of depressive disorders.

| Class | Agent | Dosages (daily) | Ages[a] (years) |
|---|---|---|---|
| Antidepressants | | | |
| Tricyclics | Imipramine | (1–2.5 mg/kg) | ≥18 |
| | Nortriptyline | (1–2 mg/kg) | ≥18 |
| | Amitriptyline | (1–2.5 mg/kg) | ≥12 |
| | Doxepin | (1–2.5 mg/kg) | ≥12 |
| MAOIs | Isocarboxazid | 5–40 mg | ≥16 |
| | Phenelzine | 7.5–45 mg | ≥16 |
| | Tranylcypromine | 5–30 mg | ≥18 |
| | Selegiline (transdermal) | 6, 9, or 12 mg[b] | ≥18 |
| SSRIs | Fluoxetine | 5–60 mg (0.25–1 mg/kg) | ≥8 |
| | Paroxetine | 5–40 mg (0.25–1 mg/kg) | ≥18 |
| | Sertraline | 12.5–200 mg (1.5–3 mg/kg) | ≥18 |
| | Citalopram | 5–40 mg | ≥18 |
| | Escitalopram | 5–20 mg | ≥18 |
| SNRIs | Venlafaxine | 37.5–225 mg (1–3 mg/kg) | ≥18 |
| | Duloxetine | 20–40 mg | ≥18 |
| Other | Trazodone | 25–300 mg (2–5 mg/kg) | ≥6 |
| | Nefazodone | 25–300 mg | ≥18 |
| | Bupropion | 75–300 mg (3–6 mg/kg) | ≥18 |
| | Mirtazapine | 7.5–45 mg | ≥18 |
| Mood stabilizers | Lithium[c] | 25–35 mg/kg/d, div. 2–3x/d | ≥12 |
| | Lamotrigine | 12.5–25 mg/d, then inc. by 25 mg q 1–2 wks | ≥18 |
| | Valproic acid[c] | 20 mg/kg/d, 2–3x/d | ≥18 |
| | Carbamazepine[c] | 7 mg/kg/d, 2–3x/d | Off-label |
| | Oxcarbazepine | 20–29 kg: 900 mg/d 30–39 kg: 1200 mg/d >39 kg: 1800 mg/d | Off-label |
| Antipsychotics | Quetiapine | 200–600 mg/d | ≥18 |
| | Olanzapine | 5–20 mg/d | ≥18 |
| Combination | OLZ/FLX (mg/mg) | 6/25, 6/50, 12/25, or 12/50 | ≥18 |

[a] FDA-approved ages for the treatment of major depressive disorder or bipolar disorder.

[b] Each patch is effective for 24 hours.

[c] Adjust dosage to achieve a therapeutic level and to avoid a toxic level.

OLZ, Olanzapine; FLX, Fluoxetine.

antidepressant use in children and adolescents. In some practice settings primary care physicians have significantly reduced the numbers of new prescriptions for antidepressants. Others have felt uncomfortable monitoring patients already on these medications, even if they remained stable and were without thoughts of suicide or self-harm. In some communities this has led either to an increase in referrals to child and adolescent psychiatrists or nontreatment of children who need to be treated with antidepressant medication.

Although the data did identify a two-fold increase in suicidal ideation in the children and adolescents being treated with antidepressants, the actual percentages were small, and there were no actual suicides. Conversely, other studies have discovered that the greatest risk for suicide is in the month before instituting pharmacotherapy, and that there is an inverse correlation between the number of antidepressants prescribed and the risk of suicide. The safe use of antidepressants will be covered in the section "How to use the medications."

(1) Selective serotonin reuptake inhibitors. The common side effects of the SSRIs are nausea, insomnia, diarrhea, rash, nervousness, agitation, and akathisia (the latter three sometimes referred to as "behavioral activation"). There is some evidence that paroxetine may cause more activation than the other SSRIs. A more serious adverse condition is the *serotonin syndrome*, which is caused by excessive CNS serotonergic activity. It is characterized by mental status changes (most notably confusion), tachycardia, hypo- or hypertension, motor abnormalities (especially muscular rigidity and myoclonus), fever and diaphoresis, and various gastrointestinal symptoms.

(2) Other (newer) classes. Although nefazodone shares many of the side effects of the SSRIs, it may also cause hepatic failure. Mirtazapine is quite sedating (especially at lower doses), frequently causes weight gain, may elevate serum cholesterol and transaminases, and may impair cognition. Bupropion can lower the seizure threshold, and can also cause agitation, anxiety, insomnia, weight loss, and tremors. Venlafaxine and duloxetine have side-effect profiles very similar to that of bupropion, but with a much lower risk of seizure activity. Venlafaxine and duloxetine may increase blood pressure. Venlafaxine may also increase serum cholesterol.

(3) Tricyclic antidepressants. The effects that the TCAs can have on the cardiovascular system can range from mild tachycardia and

hypotension to cardiac arrhythmia and heart block; these are dose-related. The use of desipramine in children has been associated with some cardiac deaths. Other side effects include dry mouth, blurred vision, constipation or diarrhea, difficulty with urination, hyperprolactinemia, hypo- or hyperglycemia, and dilutional hyponatremia.

(4) Monoamine oxidase inhibitors. The most common side effects of the MAOIs are dizziness, headache, somnolence, sleep disturbances, tremors, constipation, dry mouth, weight gain, and postural hypotension. Abnormal laboratory indices can include elevated transaminases, hypo- or hypernatremia, and leukopenia.

(5) Mood stabilizers. Lithium commonly causes increased thirst, polyuria, fine hand tremors, mild gastrointestinal upset, and leukocytosis. Serious side effects of concern include hypothyroidism, renal insufficiency, cardiac arrhythmias, electrolyte disturbances (secondary to vomiting and/or diarrhea), and lithium toxicity. The anticonvulsants can elevate transaminase levels, and valproic acid, carbamazepine, and lamotrigine have caused hepatic failure in some patients. Valproic acid may also cause thrombocytopenia and severe pancreatitis. Carbamazepine has produced agranulocytosis and aplastic anemia. Carbamazepine and oxcarbazepine may reduce the efficacy of oral contraceptives. Anticonvulsants may increase risk of suicidality (FDA, 2008).

(6) Antipsychotics (see Chapter 8 for details). These medications can cause extrapyramidal symptoms, neuroleptic malignant syndrome, hypotension, sedation, hyperprolactinemia, weight gain (especially olanzapine), hyperglycemia, and/or hyperlipidemia.

## Contraindications

(1) Selective serotonin reuptake inhibitors. As a class, the SSRIs should not be used concomitantly with the MAOIs, pimozide, or triptans. In addition, neither fluoxetine nor paroxetine should be used with thioridazine. The SSRIs should be used with extreme caution if other serotonergic agents are also being used.

(2) Other (newer) classes. Nefazodone should not be used with carbamazepine, pimozide, or MAOIs. In addition, nefazodone should not be used in patients with evidence of hepatic dysfunction. There are no specific contraindications to the use of mirtazapine; however,

the same cautions exist regarding concurrent use with MAOIs. The use of bupropion is contraindicated in patients with a seizure disorder, an eating disorder, withdrawing from a CNS depressant, or taking an MAOI. Bupropion should also be used with extreme caution in patients taking medications which may also lower the seizure threshold. Neither venlafaxine nor duloxetine should be used along with an MAOI or a triptan.

(3) Tricyclic antidepressants. The TCAs should not be used concomitantly with the MAOIs, or with medications that prolong the $QT_c$ interval. They should be used with caution in patients with a history of seizures, narrow-angle glaucoma, or thyroid supplementation.

(4) Monoamine oxidase inhibitors. The MAOIs should not be used in the presence of hepatic dysfunction. They should not be used concomitantly with other types of antidepressants, sympathomimetics, CNS depressants, buspirone, dextromethorphan, tryptophan, meperidine, or foods with high levels of tyramine.

(5) Mood stabilizers. Lithium should not be used in patients with severe cardiovascular disease, renal disease (unless having dialysis), dehydration, or sodium depletion (or on natriuretic medications). Valproic acid should not be used in the presence of significant hepatic dysfunction or a urea cycle disorder. Carbamazepine (given its tricyclic structure) should not be used with an MAOI. Its use should also be avoided in persons with a history of bone marrow suppression and in persons with acute intermittent porphyria.

(6) Antipsychotics (see Chapter 8 for details). No specific contraindications to the use of olanzapine or quetiapine.

## How to use the medications (see Figures 6.1 and 6.2)

(1) Selective serotonin reuptake inhibitors. These are the medications of choice for the treatment of child and adolescent depression. The SSRIs with the best efficacy and safety data are fluoxetine, sertraline, and citalopram. Paroxetine tends to have more side effects and withdrawal effects than the other SSRIs. Once an agent has been chosen and treatment initiated, it should be continued for at least 4 weeks before a decision is made to increase the dose or switch to a different agent. Dosage increases should occur no less frequently than every 4 weeks. The medication is increased until a positive clinical response is

**Table 6.4** Tricyclic antidepressant therapeutic levels.[a]

| | |
|---|---|
| Amitriptyline (AMI) | 120–150 ng/ml |
| Nortriptyline (NOR) | 50–150 ng/ml |
| AMI and NOR | 120–250 ng/ml |
| Imipramine (IMI) | 150–300 ng/ml |
| Desipramine (DES) | 150–300 ng/ml |
| IMI and DES | 125–225 ng/ml |

[a] Levels established for adults

obtained, intolerable (or dangerous) side effects occur, or the maximum dosage is arrived at with no, or incomplete, clinical response. Due to higher metabolic activity in children and adolescents, dosing of certain medications that are usually given once a day in adults (such as sertraline, paroxetine, and citalopram) may have to be divided into twice-daily dosing to prevent withdrawal effects. If the patient does not respond to adequate trials of two different SSRIs, the clinician may then try an agent from one of the other, newer classes of antidepressants.

(2) Other (newer) classes. Choices from this group include nefazodone, mirtazapine, venlafaxine, bupropion, and duloxetine. Some of these agents have not been studied in younger patients using a randomized, double-blind design. For those that have, results are either negative or inconclusive when compared to placebo. A trial of one of these agents should still be considered if the depression is not remitting or is getting worse. As with the other medications, starting at a low dose, titrating slowly, and allowing sufficient time for the medication to work are essential.

(3) Tricyclic antidepressants. These medications have shown only moderate efficacy in adolescent depression, and no efficacy in childhood depression, when compared with placebo. Their use, therefore, should only be considered in adolescents who have not responded to the medications noted previously. If used, the TCAs should be started at low dosages and titrated slowly, monitoring the patient's clinical status, drug plasma levels, and the ECG (the latter being more important than the drug level). Toxicity may occur even if the plasma drug level is in the therapeutic range (Table 6.4), so monitoring of the ECG for tachycardia, arrhythmias, and QRS

prolongation is important. The use of desipramine is not recommended, as it has an unfavorable risk: benefit ratio.

(4) Monoamine oxidase inhibitors. The use of MAOIs is a last medication choice before considering ECT. To avoid the serotonin syndrome, at least 2 weeks should be allowed after stopping an SSRI (1 week for venlafaxine and bupropion) before starting an MAOI; for fluoxetine, given its long half-life, at least 5 weeks should be allowed after stopping it before starting an MAOI. Conversely, other antidepressants should not be started within 14 days of discontinuing therapy with an MAOI. The patient and parents/guardians should be educated about avoiding high tyramine-content foods and certain prescription and over-the-counter medications (detailed information can be found in the medication package inserts, or obtained from the pharmacist or on-line). These restrictions do not appear to be necessary if the lowest dose (6 mg/24 hour) selegiline patch is used.

(5) Mood stabilizers. As noted previously, these medications are used to augment the effects of antidepressants for the treatment of MDD (Figure 6.1) or to treat bipolar depression (Figure 6.2). Dosing ranges and schedules are noted in Table 6.3; monitoring recommendations are described in the section "How to monitor the medication" that follows.

(6) Antipsychotics. As noted previously, these medications are used to treat the psychosis that may occur with severe MDD (Chapter 8 addresses the treatment of schizophrenia and other psychotic disorders). They may also be used to treat bipolar depression (Figure 6.2). The lowest dosage to achieve good clinical response should be used, and the patient should be monitored closely for side effects (see below).

## How to monitor the medication

(1) Selective serotonin reuptake inhibitors. Clinical monitoring only; no specific laboratory testing is required.

(2) Other (newer) classes. Although no laboratory testing is recommended for mirtazapine use, in younger patients it would be wise to periodically check serum cholesterol and transaminase levels. Blood pressure should be routinely checked in patients taking venlafaxine or

duloxetine. A yearly serum cholesterol level should be considered in patients taking venlafaxine.

(3) Tricyclic antidepressants. An ECG should be obtained at baseline, during dosage titration, and after subsequent increases in dosage. Check blood glucose and serum sodium levels periodically. Check serum prolactin if gynecomastia or menstrual irregularities appear. Check liver function tests if unexplained gastrointestinal symptoms are present.

(4) Monoamine oxidase inhibitors. Blood pressure should be checked at baseline and during dosage increases, and any time there is a complaint about headache or palpitations. Check liver function tests and serum sodium levels periodically.

(5) Mood stabilizers. For lithium, baseline electrolytes, BUN, creatinine, thyroid function tests, WBC, and urine specific gravity are recommended. These labs should be repeated 1–2 times/year when the patient is stable. A serum lithium trough level (10–12 hours after last dose) should be measured 4–5 days after starting the medication, 4–5 days after any dosage increase, and every 3–6 months during the maintenance phase. For patients on valproic acid, baseline and follow-up (every 6–12 months) liver function tests and CBC should be obtained. The valproate drug level should be checked 1–2 weeks after initiation or after each dosage increase, and also every 3–6 months during maintenance. The monitoring for carbamazepine is similar to that for valproic acid.

(6) Antipsychotics (see Chapter 8 for details). The patient's height, weight, BMI, blood pressure, and pulse should be measured before starting antipsychotic medications and at each subsequent visit. Fasting glucose and lipid levels should be measured before starting treatment, 3 months afterwards, and then every 6 months thereafter. The patient should be examined for extrapyramidal symptoms before and after starting antipsychotic medications. Prolactin levels should be checked if menstrual abnormalities or sexual problems develop.

## ■ Summary

Most of the algorithms for the treatment of MDD have been developed for use in adults. This chapter contains our recommendations for the treatment

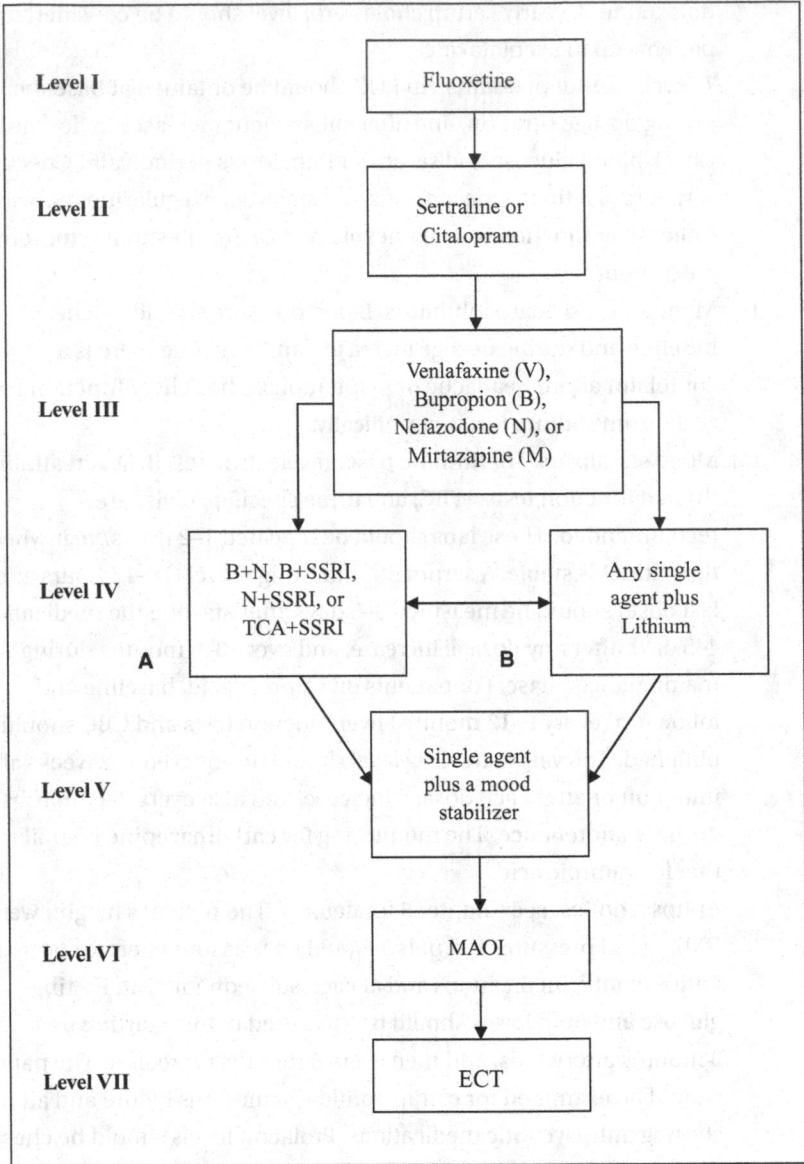

**Figure 6.1** Treatment algorithm for major depressive disorder without psychosis.

of MDD without psychosis (Figure 6.1) and bipolar depression without psychosis (Figure 6.2) in younger patients. The change from one treatment level to the next is based on nonresponse or poor response to the medication(s) at the preceding level.

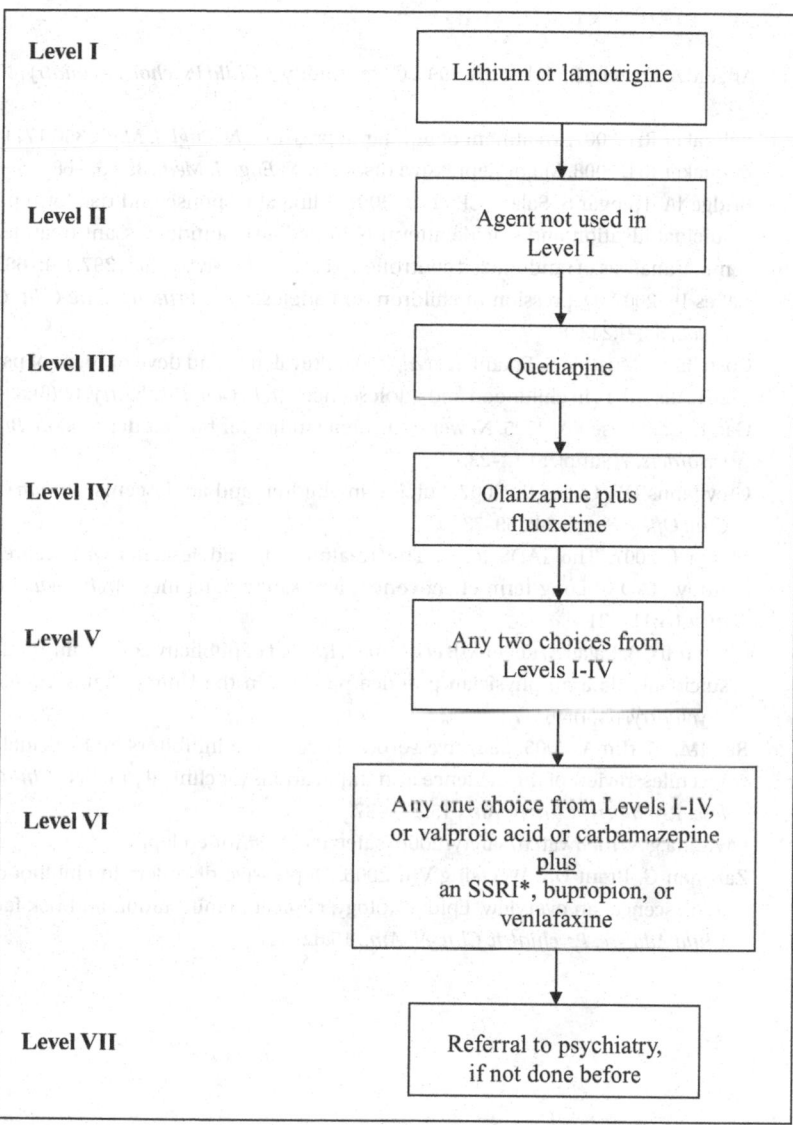

**Figure 6.2** Treatment algorithm for bipolar depression. (*Other than fluoxetine).

Angold A, Costello EJ, Erkanli A. 1999. Comorbidity. *J. Child Psychol. Psychiatry*, 40:57–87.

Belmaker RH. 2007. Treatment of bipolar depression, *N. Engl. J. Med.*, 356:1771–3.

Belmaker RH. 2008. Major depressive disorder. *N. Engl. J. Med.*, 358:55–68.

Bridge JA, Iyengar S, Salary CB *et al.* 2007. Clinical response and risk for reported suicidal ideation and suicide attempts in pediatric antidepressant treatment. A meta-analysis of randomized controlled trials. *J. Am. Med. Assoc.*, 297(15):1683–96.

Calles JL. 2007. Depression in children and adolescents. *Primary Care Clin. Office Pract.*, 33(2):243–8.

Costello EJ, Mustillo S, Erkanli A *et al.* 2003. Prevalence and development of psychiatric disorders in childhood and adolescence. *Arch. Gen. Psychiatry*, 60(8):837–44.

Gao K, Calabrese KA. 2005. Newer treatment studies for bipolar depression. *Bipolar Disorders*, 7(Suppl. 5):13–23.

Greydanus DE, Calles JL. 2007. Suicide in children and adolescents. *Primary Care Clin. Office Pract.*, 34:259–73.

March J. 2007. The TADS team. The treatment for adolescents with depression study (TADS): Long-term effectiveness and safety outcomes. *Arch. Gen. Psychiatry*, 64:111–21.

Nemeroff CB, Kalali A, Keller MB *et al.* 2007. Impact of publicity concerning pediatric suicidality data on physician practice patterns in the United States. *Arch. Gen. Psychiatry*, 64(4):466–72.

Rey JM, Martin A. 2006. Selective serotonin reuptake inhibitors and suicidality in juveniles: review of the evidence and implications for clinical practice. *Child Adolesc. Psychiatric Clin. N. Am.*, 15:221–37.

www.fda.gov/medwatch/safety/2008/safety08.htm#Antiepileptic

Zalsman G, Brent DA, Weersing VR. 2006. Depressive disorders in childhood and adolescence: an overview. Epidemiology, clinical manifestation and risk factors. *Child Adolesc. Psychiatric Clin. N. Am.*, 15:827–41.

# Disruptive behavior and aggressive disorders

## 7

Children and adolescents with behavioral disturbances commonly come to the attention of primary care physicians. Although disruptive behaviors can be associated with any number of psychiatric disorders, this chapter will focus on three diagnoses wherein behavioral symptoms are key diagnostic criteria: oppositional defiant disorder (ODD), conduct disorder (CD), and intermittent explosive disorder (IED). A fourth diagnosis, attention-deficit/hyperactivity disorder (ADHD), is usually included in the disruptive behavior disorder (DBD) category, but will not be included in this chapter (see Chapter 4 for details about the treatment of ADHD).

## ■ Definition

The disorders covered in this chapter are considered *disruptive*, in that individuals diagnosed with them evidence behaviors that have a negative effect on their immediate environment and elicit negative responses from others. A common element of the negative behavior is *aggression*, which can be verbal or physical. Verbal aggression includes loud, profane, or threatening speech that intimidates others. Physical aggression includes damage to property or person, the latter also known as *violence*. Violent behavior exists in two basic forms: *proactive* aggression, which is premeditated and fairly dispassionate; *reactive* aggression is impulsive and affectively driven. The distinction between proactive and reactive aggression is an important one, since it is the reactive type that tends to respond to pharmacotherapy.

The disruptive aspect of ODD comes from the conflict that the individual has with rules and authority figures. Legal problems associated with ODD are relatively minor, e.g. truancy and running away. The symptoms of CD exist at another level of disruption, with major violations of societal norms and major disregard for boundaries of property and person. Legal problems associated with CD are more serious, e.g. robbery or rape, and often lead to involvement in the legal system, including incarceration. Individuals with IED have problems that are episodic and associated with intense anger outbursts ("rage"); their legal problems are usually limited to destruction of property and assault.

## ■ Epidemiology

The lifetime prevalence of ODD in the USA is about 8.5% in the general population, with symptoms usually obvious before the age of 8 years. The lifetime prevalence of CD is about 9.5% (12% among males and about 7% among females), and the median age of onset is around 11.5 years. Lifetime prevalence estimates of IED in the general population are about 7% versus about 5%, depending on whether broad or narrow diagnostic criteria, respectively, are used. The mean age of onset of the first major anger attack is somewhere between 14 and 15 years, although much younger ages are not uncommon in clinical settings.

## ■ Differential diagnosis/comorbidity

Angry and irritable moods, as well as disruptive, aggressive, or violent behaviors are often not diagnoses in their own right, but signs and symptoms of underlying medical, substance-related, or psychiatric disorders. Table 7.1 lists the diagnoses to consider when evaluating patients with disruptive and aggressive behaviors; references are also given to other chapters in this book for more details.

## ■ Psychopharmacology

Table 7.2 lists the pharmacologic classes and agents which may be used to treat disruptive and aggressive behavior disorders. Recommendations for use in specific problem areas will be described in the section "How to use the medications."

**Table 7.1** Disorders associated with disruptive behaviors and aggression.

*Medical*
Seizure disorders
Traumatic brain injury
Encephalitis/meningitis
Sensory impairments
Huntington's disease
Wilson's disease
Lafora's disease
Acute intermittent porphyria
Hartnup's disease
Neuroacanthocytosis
Developmental disorders (see Chapter 10)

*Substance-related* (see Chapter 13)
Alcohol abuse/dependence: Intoxication or withdrawal
Anxiolytic abuse/dependence: Intoxication or withdrawal
Cannabis abuse/dependence: Withdrawal
Stimulant abuse/dependence: Intoxication

*Psychiatric*
Attention-deficit/hyperactivity disorder (see Chapter 5)
Oppositional defiant disorder
Conduct disorder
Intermittent explosive disorder
Mental retardation (see Chapter 10)
Autistic spectrum disorders (see Chapter 9)
Language disorders
Mood disorders (see Chapter 4):
   Major depressive disorder
   Bipolar disorder
Anxiety disorders (see Chapter 3):
   Post-traumatic stress disorder
   Social anxiety disorder
   Separation anxiety disorder
Psychotic disorders (see Chapter 8)
Tic disorders (see Chapter 12)
Personality disorders
   Borderline personality disorder (mostly females)
   Antisocial personality disorder (mostly males)
   Paranoid personality disorder (mostly males)

**Table 7.2** Medications used to treat disruptive and aggressive behavior disorders, and ages at which use may be appropriate.[a]

| Class | Agent | Doses[a] | Ages[b] |
|---|---|---|---|
| Psychostimulants: See Chapter 5 for details | | | |
| Antidepressants: See Chapter 6 for details | | | |
| Anxiolytics: See Chapter 4 for details | | | |
| **Alpha-agonists** | Clonidine | 0.05–0.20, 2–3×/d | ≥12 |
| **Antipsychotics** | | | |
| *First-generation* | | | |
| Phenothiazines | Chlorpromazine | 50–400 mg/d | ≥1[b] |
| | Thioridazine | 50–400 mg/d | ≥2[b] |
| Butyrophenones | Haloperidol | 2–10 mg/d | ≥3[b] |
| *Second-generation* | Risperidone | 1–4 mg/d | ≥18 |
| | Olanzapine | 5–20 mg/d | ≥18 |
| | Quetiapine | 200–600 mg/d | ≥18 |
| | Ziprasidone | 80–120 mg/d | ≥18 |
| **Mood stabilizers** | | | |
| Lithium salts | Lithium carbonate | 25–35 mg/kg/d, div. 2–3x/d (adj. to level) | ≥12 |
| Anticonvulsants | Carbamazepine | 7 mg/kg/d, 2–3×/d (adj. to level) | Any (?) |
| | Valproic acid | 20 mg/kg/d, 2–3×/d (adj. to level) | ≥10 |
| | Oxcarbazepine | **20–29 kg**: 900 mg/d **30–39 kg**: 1200 mg/d **>39 kg**: 1800 mg/d | ≥18 |
| **Beta-blockers** | Propranolol | **<35 kg**: 10–20 mg; **>35 kg**: 20–40 mg, both at 2×/d dosing | |
| | Metoprolol | 12.5–25 mg, 2×/d | ≥18 (all) |
| | Pindolol | 6.25–12.5 mg, 2×/d | |
| | Nadolol | 5–10 mg, 1×/d | |

[a] Dosing is clinically based, unless stated otherwise.

[b] Ages (years) are for FDA-approved indications; use for other indications and/or at other ages is based on clinical judgement.

# Medication classification and mechanism of action

## Psychostimulants

The amphetamines are non-catecholamine, sympathomimetic amines that act as powerful CNS stimulants. Their putative mechanism of action involves reuptake blockade of neurotransmitters (dopamine and nor-epinephrine) into presynaptic neurons, as well as an increased release of those neurotransmitters into the synaptic cleft. Methylphenidate, a non-amphetamine sympathomimetic, acts as a mild CNS stimulant; its mechanism of action is believed to be mediated through activation of brain stem and cortical arousal systems. Atomoxetine, a nonstimulant used to treat ADHD, is discussed with the antidepressants.

## Antidepressants

Although the precise mechanisms through which these agents exert their clinical effects are unknown, their efficacy is hypothesized to be related to an increase of available catecholamine neurotransmitters in the CNS. Therapeutic changes occur via downregulation of postsynaptic neurons. The MAO inhibitors (MAOI) prevent the breakdown of the monoamine neurotransmitters present in presynaptic neurons. The tricyclic antidepressants (TCAs) block reuptake of all the catecholamine neurotransmitters into presynaptic neurons. The selective serotonin reuptake inhibitors (SSRIs) selectively block the reuptake of serotonin into presynaptic neurons. Atomoxetine, although used to treat ADHD, is essentially an antidepressant, in that its mechanism of action relies on selective inhibition of norepinephrine reuptake. Antidepressants in other classes exert their effects through reuptake inhibition, pre- and/or postsynaptic antagonism, or a combination.

## Anxiolytics

Benzodiazepines bind to specific receptors in the CNS, especially in the limbic system and other deep-brain structures, producing the calming effect that these medications are known for. Buspirone, a nonbenzodiazepine anxiolytic, may produce its calming effects through $5HT_{1A}$ receptor binding.

## Alpha-agonists

These agents stimulate brainstem $alpha_2$-adrenoreceptors, effectively reducing CNS sympathetic outflow. As the sympathetic nervous system is involved in the "fight or flight" response, the alpha-agonists may serve to blunt anxiety or aggression in some individuals.

## Antipsychotics

The hypothesized mechanism of action for these medications is related to their ability to antagonize dopamine receptors. Regarding the "atypical" or second-generation antipsychotics (SGAs), an additional action may be derived via serotonin receptor antagonism.

## Mood stabilizers

Lithium affects neuronal sodium transport, which may affect how nerve cells process catecholamines; how this contributes to its anti-manic or anti-aggressive effects is unclear. The numerous available anticonvulsants likely have different mechanisms by which they exert their effects. Proposed theories include neuronal membrane stabilization, the inhibition of excitatory amino acids (e.g. glutamate and aspartate), and the increase of gamma amino-butyric acid (GABA), a known inhibitory neurotransmitter.

## Beta-blockers

These agents block beta-adrenergic receptors, effectively reducing sympathetic nervous system activity. It is not known how they exert their effects in the CNS, as agents vary by degree of selectivity for beta$_1$ (mostly cardiac) and beta$_2$ (noncardiac) receptors, and also vary in degree of lipophilia (propranolol, pindolol, and metoprolol are quite lipid-soluble; nadolol is more water-soluble).

## Side-effects (adverse effects)

### Psychostimulants

Observed adverse reactions include bland facial expression, decreased social interactions, and impaired cognition. The stimulants can provoke or increase irritability, psychomotor activity (including tics), and anxiety. Insomnia may be produced or exacerbated by stimulant use. These medications commonly reduce appetite and can also lead to loss of body weight, and in some patients may prevent them from achieving their full height potential.

## Antidepressants

The SSRIs can cause agitation, akathisia, and hypomania (especially in those at risk for bipolar disorder). Another concern with the SSRIs is the serotonin syndrome, especially when they are used concomitantly with other serotonergic agents. Bupropion can lower the seizure threshold. With the exception of bupropion and mirtazapine, all of the commonly used antidepressants can cause hyponatremia and/or SIADH. Atomoxetine commonly causes headache and stomach upset, may increase blood pressure and heart rate, and can cause irritability and mood instability.

## Anxiolytics

The benzodiazepines can cause sedation, behavioral disinhibition (similar to that seen with alcohol intoxication), worsening of cognitive functioning, and withdrawal seizures. They also have the potential for being abused or causing dependence. The use of buspirone avoids the abuse and dependence issues, but not the side effects.

## Alpha-agonists

Common side effects include dry mouth, drowsiness, dizziness, constipation, and sedation. Children generally experience orthostatic hypotension less than adults do; however, children may be more susceptible to rebound hypertension if these agents are discontinued abruptly.

## Antipsychotics

Adverse effects from these agents include hyperglycemia, hyperlipidemia, hyperprolactinemia, extrapyramidal symptoms (EPS), and weight gain. As treatment with antipsychotics may need to be long term in some cases, the possible development of tardive dyskinesia is a serious concern.

## Mood stabilizers

Common lithium side effects include increased thirst, polyuria, fine resting hand tremors, mild gastrointestinal upset, and leukocytosis. More serious associated conditions include hypothyroidism, renal insufficiency, cardiac arrhythmias, diarrhea with electrolyte disturbances, and lithium toxicity (with significant neurologic signs and symptoms).

All of the anticonvulsants used as mood stabilizers can elevate liver function tests values. They have also been associated with Stevens–Johnson syndrome and toxic epidermal necrolyis. Hepatic failure has been reported with valproic acid and carbamazepine. Valproic acid can cause life-threatening pancreatitis; it can also cause thrombocytopenia. Aplastic anemia and agranulocytosis have been reported with carbamazepine. Carbamazepine and oxcarbazepine may reduce the efficacy of oral contraceptives. Anticonvulsants increase the risk of suicidal thoughts and depression (FDA, 2008).

## Beta-blockers

Common side effects include dizziness, fatigue, bradycardia, mental status changes, gastrointestinal upset, and various skin rashes. Less common – but more serious – adverse events can be bronchospasm and heart failure, both of which may occur more readily in children.

## Contraindications

### Psychostimulants

These medications are contraindicated in patients who are already experiencing significant levels of anxiety, inner tension, or psychomotor agitation. They should not be used if glaucoma is present. They should also not be used if patients are on MAOIs, inhibitors, or if those medications have been discontinued within the last 2 weeks. Their use in the presence of motor tic disorder or Tourette's disorder is relatively contraindicated (see Chapter 12). Another relative contraindication is a seizure disorder. The use of the mixed amphetamines is also contraindicated if the patient has symptomatic cardiovascular disease, hypertension, or hyperthyroidism.

### Antidepressants

All of the non-MAOI antidepressants (and atomoxetine) are contraindicated for concurrent use with MAOIs, or if an MAOI has been discontinued within the previous 2 weeks. Before starting an MAOI, most other antidepressants should be stopped at least 2 weeks beforehand (venlafaxine requires at least 1 week; fluoxetine requires at least 5 weeks). All antidepressants with serotonergic activity (except mirtazapine and venlafaxine) are contraindicated for use with pimozide, the combination of which can greatly prolong the $QT_c$ interval (fluoxetine and paroxetine should not be used concurrently with thioridazine, and nefazodone with carbamazepine, for similar reasons).

Bupropion is contraindicated in patients with a seizure disorder or an eating disorder (which, in combination with bupropion, increases the risk of a seizure).

The MAOI antidepressants should not be used in patients with pheochromocytoma, heart failure or other cardiovascular disease, cerebrovascular disease, or liver disease. There are also several medications which should not be used in combination with the MAOIs, especially dextromethorphan, meperidine, and any with sympathomimetic actions.

Atomoxetine should not be used in patients with narrow angle glaucoma.

## Anxiolytics

The benzodiazepines should not be used if patients have acute narrow angle glaucoma. Abuse or dependence potential may exclude use in certain individuals. The use of buspirone is contraindicated in combination with an MAOI.

## Alpha-agonists

There are no known specific contraindications to their use, although hypotension may preclude their use in certain individuals.

## Antipsychotics

The older, first-generation antipsychotics (FGA) are contraindicated in patients with blood dyscrasias, hepatic damage, subcortical brain damage, and obtundation. The use of thioridazine is also contraindicated in patients with congenital long $QT_c$ syndrome, who are taking other medications that can prolong the $QT_c$ interval, or who already have cardiac arrhythmias.

The SGAs, as a group, do not carry any specific contraindications, with some exceptions. The cautions about potential cardiac arrhythmias during the use of ziprasidone are similar to those associated with thioridazine.

## Mood stabilizers

Lithium should not be used in patients with severe cardiovascular disease, renal disease (unless already on dialysis), dehydration, or sodium depletion (or medications that cause it). Persons with brain damage may be more sensitive to lithium's neurotoxic potential.

Given that carbamazepine has a tricyclic structure, its use with MAOI needs to follow the same guidelines as noted previously for the antidepressants. It should be avoided in persons with prior bone marrow suppression, as well as in individuals with acute intermittent porphyria. Although oxcarbazepine is very closely related to carbamazepine, it does not have specific restrictions to its use (other than known hypersensitivity to the drug itself).

Valproic acid should not be used in the presence of significant hepatic dysfunction or a urea cycle disorder.

## Beta-blockers

These medications should not be used in patients with sinus bradycardia and greater than first-degree heart block, asthma, sick sinus syndrome, significant peripheral arterial disease, pheochromocytoma, and right ventricular failure associated with pulmonary hypertension.

## How to use the medications

If a patient's disruptive/aggressive behavior is felt to be secondary to a specific psychiatric disorder, treatment for that disorder should proceed in a manner that will have the best chance of relieving all symptoms, including the behavioral ones. Recommendations for medications are listed in Table 7.3, and are discussed below. For the treatment of any disorder, if none of the interventions are effective or tolerated, a re-evaluation of the patient should be undertaken, looking for previously missed comorbid diagnoses or even a misdiagnosis. The clinician has the option of referring the patient to a psychiatrist at any point during the treatment process.

## Psychostimulants

The disruptive behaviors in a child with ADHD may often improve, or even resolve, if the ADHD itself is properly treated. The stimulant medications should be used cautiously, however, as they may provoke irritability and aggression in some individuals. If a trial of a stimulant – methylphenidate or mixed-amphetamine salts – is ineffective or worsens the behavior, a second trial with the stimulant not previously used is indicated. If neither stimulant is effective, or if they especially exacerbate the behavioral symptoms, then a trial of either clonidine or a beta-blocker (preferably the former) should be tried (see their respective sections below). How the medications are dosed is important. The longer-acting stimulants are preferred, as the wearing

**Table 7.3** Disorders associated with aggressive or violent behaviors, and recommended pharmacotherapeutic strategies.

| Disorder | Medications | | |
| --- | --- | --- | --- |
| | First-line | Second-line | Third-line |
| ADHD | Stimulant | 2nd stimulant | Alpha-agonist or beta-blocker |
| Anxiety | SSRI | 2nd SSRI or alpha-agonist | Buspirone |
| ASD ± MR | Risperidone | 2nd SGA | AED |
| Bipolar disorder | Lithium | VPA or CBZ | 2nd AED or an SGA |
| Conduct disorder | Lithium | SGA | Chlorpromazine |
| Depression | Fluoxetine | 2nd SSRI | Non-SSRI AD or lithium |
| IED | Lithium | AED | SGA |
| Psychosis | SGA | 2nd SGA | 3rd SGA or an FGA |
| TBI | Alpha-agonist or beta-blocker | AED | SSRI |

ADHD, attention-deficit/hyperactivity disorder; ASD, autistic-spectrum disorder; MR, mental retardation; IED, intermittent explosive disorder; TBI, traumatic brain injury; AD, antidepressant; AED, antiepileptic drug; CBZ, carbamazepine; FGA, first-generation antipsychotic; SGA, second-generation antipsychotic; SSRI, selective serotonin reuptake inhibitor; VPA, valproic acid.

off of the shorter-acting stimulants is more likely to produce agitation and irritability.

## Antidepressants

For depression, fluoxetine is the clear choice for first agent to use. As noted previously, the patient's lack of, or adverse, reaction to fluoxetine would dictate a second medication trial with another SSRI. If that agent also is ineffective or exacerbates the behavioral symptoms, then a third trial, this time with a non-SSRI antidepressant (except for bupropion) or with lithium, should be initiated.

For anxiety, treatment can start with any SSRI, followed by a second SSRI (if the first was ineffective or poorly tolerated) or an alpha-agonist. If neither of the second-line medications are effective, an anxiolytic should be considered (see below).

## Anxiolytics

The recommended agent for the combination of anxiety and aggression (not responsive to other agents – see above) is buspirone. Dosing needs to be on a 3 times a day schedule, to compensate for the higher metabolic activity in younger people, and to prevent rebound anxiety and agitation.

## Alpha-agonists

Clonidine is a versatile agent. As discussed above, it is a third-line agent for use in patients with ADHD-associated aggression, and a second-line agent for aggression associated with anxiety. Along with the beta-blockers (see the discussion below), clonidine is a first-choice treatment for the aggression associated with traumatic brain injury. Dosing should be at least twice-daily to avoid rebound symptomatology (clonidine is short-acting).

## Antipsychotics

The use of these agents for aggression associated with psychosis essentially follows the standard protocol for treatment of schizophrenia (see Chapter 8). Risperidone is the drug of choice for the agitation and aggression associated with autistic spectrum disorders (the other second-generation antipsychotics (SGAs) can be used as second-line agents). Any of the SGAs can be used as third-line agents for the aggression associated with conduct disorder or bipolar disorder. The first-generation antipsychotic (FGA) chlorpromazine can be used as a third-line agent to treat the disruptive behaviors associated with conduct disorder.

## Mood stabilizers

Lithium is the treatment of choice for the aggression seen in patients with bipolar disorder, conduct disorder, and intermittent explosive disorder. As mentioned previously, lithium is also a third-line agent for depression-associated aggression. The anticonvulsants valproic acid and carbamazepine are second-line agents for bipolar disorder with marked behavioral disturbances. The anticonvulsant mood stabilizers are second-line agents for treating the aggression in intermittent explosive disorder and the disruptive behavior in patients with traumatic brain injury. They are also used as third-line agents in autistic spectrum disorders and bipolar disorder.

## Beta-blockers

These agents can be used, instead of alpha-agonists, as first-line agents to treat the aggression associated with traumatic brain injury, or as third-line agents to control disruptive behaviors associated with ADHD.

## How to monitor the medications

### Psychostimulants

In cases of chronic treatment, periodic complete blood count (CBC), with differential and platelet count, are recommended. Blood pressure and pulse should be checked at each medication visit, as both values can increase with stimulant treatment. Height and weight should be measured per routine schedule, and any significant slowing, stoppage, or loss should prompt discontinuation and medical evaluation.

### Antidepressants

No routine laboratory tests are required for any of these medications. However, venlafaxine may raise serum cholesterol, such that checking levels should be considered during prolonged treatment. The selegiline patch infrequently elevates liver function test values; routine testing is not recommended. For patients on atomoxetine pulse and blood pressure should be measured at baseline, following dose increases, and periodically during treatment.

### Anxiolytics

For patients on long-term therapy with a benzodiazepine, periodic blood testing of the WBC (to check for neutropenia) and liver function tests (to check for elevated bilirubin or LDH) are advised.

### Alpha-agonists

Blood pressure should be monitored for hypotension and rebound hypertension. No laboratory studies are required.

## Antipsychotics

It is important that the patient's height, weight, body-mass index, blood pressure, pulse, and fasting glucose and lipids be measured before starting treatment with these agents. A baseline examination for extrapyramidal signs is suggested. The only atypical antipsychotic that requires baseline and follow-up ECGs is ziprasidone. All of these parameters, as well as a serum prolactin level (especially in females), should be rechecked during the course of treatment.

## Mood stabilizers

Before starting lithium obtain baseline electrolytes, BUN, creatinine, thyroid function tests, WBC, and urine specific gravity; repeat 1 or 2 times/year, once the patient is stabilized. A serum lithium trough level (10–12 hours after last dose) should be measured 4–5 days after starting the medication, 4–5 days after any dosage increase, and every 3–6 months during the maintenance phase.

In patients on valproic acid, baseline and follow-up (every 6–12 months) AST, ALT, LDH, and CBC should be measured. The drug level should be checked 1–2 weeks after initiation or after each dosage increase, and also every 3–6 months during maintenance.

The monitoring for carbamazepine is essentially the same as for valproic acid.

## Beta-blockers

Blood pressure and pulse should be routinely monitored. There is rarely a need for laboratory testing for these medications. Propranolol can sometimes cause elevations in serum potassium, AST, ALT, and alkaline phosphatase in hypertensive patients. Pindolol can also occasionally elevate AST, ALT, and alkaline phosphatase, as well as LDH and uric acid.

SELECTED BIBLIOGRAPHY

Calles, JL. 2006. Psychopharmacology for the violent adolescent. *Primary Care. Clin Office Pract.*, 33:531–44.
Gosalakkal JA. 2003. Aggression, rage and dyscontrol in neurological diseases of children. *J. Pediatr. Neurol.*, 1(1):9–14.

Kessler RC, Coccaro EF, Fava M, Jaeger S, Jin R, Walters E. 2006. The prevalence and correlates of DSM-IV Intermittent Explosive Disorder in the National Comorbidity Survey Replication. *Arch. Gen. Psychiatry*, 63:669–78.

Nock MK, Kazdin AE, Hiripi E, Kessler RC. 2006. Prevalence, subtypes, and correlates of DSM-IV conduct disorder in the National Comorbidity Survey Replication. *Psychol. Med.*, 36(5):699–710. Epub 2006 Jan 26.

Olvera RL. 2002. Intermittent explosive disorder: epidemiology, diagnosis and management. *CNS Drugs*, 16(8):517–26.

www.fda.gov/medwatch/safety/2008/safety08.htm#Antiepileptic

# Schizophrenia in childhood and adolescence

8

## ■ Definition

Schizophrenia is a chronic mental illness that is characterized by the presence of a formal thought disorder and associated disturbances of mood and behavior. The hallmark of the illness is a variable combination of hallucinations, delusions, disorganization, and *negative symptoms* (e.g. flat affect, poverty of thought, lack of motivation). Many other symptoms are attributed to different pathways. The age of onset of schizophrenia is typically in early adulthood, but less commonly can occur during childhood. Early-onset schizophrenia (EOS) is defined as the illness beginning before the age of 18 years; childhood-onset schizophrenia (COS; also called very-early-onset schizophrenia, or VEOS) begins before the age of 13 years.

The course of schizophrenia is quite variable, and is dependent on numerous factors. However, it has been consistently demonstrated that the earlier the onset, the poorer the outcome. Patients with EOS (and especially those with COS) tend to be male, have poor premorbid functioning (including at school), more negative symptomatology, more cognitive impairment or other developmental disabilities, stronger family history, and more obvious abnormalities on neuroimaging.

The goal of this chapter is to help the clinician to make informed decisions regarding the pharmacologic treatment of patients with this severe and chronic illness.

**Table 8.1** Differential diagnosis of psychotic symptoms.

Psychotic disorder due to a GMC or substance-induced
Delirium due to a GMC or substance-induced
Dementia due to a GMC or substance-induced
Mood disorder with psychotic features
Schizoaffective disorder
Schizophreniform disorder
Brief psychotic disorder
Delusional disorder
Psychotic disorder NOS
Pervasive developmental disorder
Communication disorder
Schizoid, schizotypal, or paranoid personality disorder

GMC, General medical condition; NOS, Not otherwise specified.

# ■ Epidemiology

Schizophrenia occurs worldwide, with adult prevalence in the range of 1% ± 0.5%. The median age of onset of the first psychotic "break" is in the early twenties for men, late twenties for women. Prevalence numbers are harder to arrive at for younger people, but for EOS estimates are that it occurs in about 1 out of every 10 000 children and adolescents, and for COS about 1 out of every 40 000 children.

# ■ Differential diagnosis/comorbidity

As schizophrenia is such a serious psychiatric disorder, it is extremely important to accurately identify and treat it as soon as possible. Some caution must be exercised, however, as there are conditions which may present with psychosis and schizophrenia-like features (see Table 8.1). Misdiagnosis could be just as harmful as missing the diagnosis, delaying appropriate treatment and possibly worsening the prognosis.

Persons with schizophrenia are at higher risk for other psychiatric disorders, including mood disorders (especially depression), anxiety disorders (especially obsessive-compulsive disorder and panic disorder), phobias, and substance-use disorders. Even in the absence of clearly identifiable comorbid diagnoses, patients with schizophrenia commonly have problems with sleep, nutrition, self-care, anger control, and suicidal ideation. (Please refer to the relevant chapters in this book for details.)

# ■ Psychopharmacology

There is a large body of literature on the psychopharmacologic treatment of schizophrenia, but the majority of it focuses on adult patients. Current use of medications for COS and EOS is either extrapolated from adult studies, or is based on case reports, open-label studies, or controlled studies with small numbers of patients. The rarity of EOS, and especially COS, makes it difficult to collect sufficient numbers of subjects for treatment studies. Research is further limited by ethical concerns regarding the use of psychotropic medications in younger people. Another hurdle is the high rate of psychiatric comorbidity in the schizophrenic population.

Table 8.2 lists the pharmacologic classes and agents which may be used in treating schizophrenia and associated conditions. Recommendations for use in specific problem areas will be described in the section "How to use the medications."

## Medication classification and mechanism of action (see Table 3.1 in Chapter 3)

### Antipsychotics

As the name implies, this category of medication is used to treat psychosis, the core disturbance in schizophrenia. There are currently available antipsychotic medications from three different classes: first-generation antipsychotics (FGA); second-generation antipsychotics (SGA); and partial dopamine agonists. Pimozide, although usually included in the antipsychotic category, will not be discussed here, as its only approved indication is for Tourette's syndrome (see Chapter 12).

The classic FGAs, of which chlorpromazine was the first, are believed to work through their potent antagonism at the dopamine $D_2$ receptor. As there are $D_2$ receptors throughout the CNS, FGA-related blockade in one pathway (mesolimbic) contributes to a desirable decrease of "positive" symptoms (hallucinations, delusions, hostility), but tends to increase many undesirable symptoms via other pathways (Table 8.3).

The SGAs have variable degrees of $D_2$ receptor blockade. In addition, they are antagonistic at serotonergic 5-$HT_2$ receptors, which may explain their lower incidence of extrapyramidal symptoms (EPS) and improvement of negative symptoms.

**Table 8.2** Medications used in persons with schizophrenia and comorbid conditions, and ages at which use may be appropriate.

| Class | Agent | Doses$^a$ (CPZ-E) | Ages$^b$ |
|---|---|---|---|
| Antipsychotics | | | |
| *First-generation* | | | |
| Phenothiazines | Chlorpromazine | 50–400 mg/d (100) | $\geq$18; 1–12$^c$ |
| | Thioridazine | 50–400 mg/d (100) | $\geq$18; $\geq$2$^c$ |
| | Fluphenazine | 2–10 mg/d (2) | $\geq$18 |
| | Perphenazine | 5–40 mg/d (10) | $\geq$18 |
| | Trifluoperazine | 2–20 mg/d (5) | $\geq$18 |
| Butyrophenones | Haloperidol | 2–10 mg/d (2) | $\geq$18; $\geq$3$^c$ |
| Miscellaneous | Loxapine | 5–50 mg/d (10) | $\geq$18 |
| | Molindone | 5–50 mg/d (10) | $\geq$18 |
| | Thiothixene | 2–20 mg/d (5) | $\geq$18 |
| *Second-generation* | Clozapine | 75–400 mg/d (30–50) | $\geq$18 |
| | Risperidone | 1–4 mg/d (2) | $\geq$13 |
| | Olanzapine | 5–20 mg/d (5) | $\geq$18 |
| | Quetiapine | 200–600 mg/d (75) | $\geq$18 |
| | Ziprasidone | 80–120 mg/d (60) | $\geq$18 |
| *Partial DA agonist* | Aripiprazole | 10–25 mg/d (7.5) | $\geq$13 |
| Anticholinergics | Benztropine | 0.5–2 mg, 1–2$\times$/d | $\geq$3 |
| | Trihexyphenidyl | 0.5–1 mg, 2–3$\times$/d | $\geq$18 |
| | Glycopyrrolate | 0.5–1 mg, 2–3$\times$/d | $\geq$18 |
| Antihistamines | Diphenhydramine | 6–11 yr: 12.5–25 mg every 4–6 hours | $\geq$6 |
| | | $\geq$12 yr: 25–50 mg every 4–6 hours | |

Beta-blockers: See Chapter 7 for details

Anxiolytics: See Chapter 4 for details

Mood stabilizers: See Chapter 7 for details

Antidepressants: See Chapter 6 for details

Sedative-hypnotics: See Chapter 11 for details

$^a$ Dosing is clinically based, unless stated otherwise.

$^b$ Ages (years) are for FDA-approved indications (see Table 3.1, Chapter 3, for details); use for other indications and/or at other ages is based on clinical judgement.

$^c$ For "severe behavioral problems."

CPZ-E, chlorpromazine equivalents, in milligrams (see the text for details). DA, Dopamine.

**Table 8.3** Antipsychotic effects on the CNS.

| CNS pathway | Effects of dopamine blockade |
|---|---|
| Mesolimbic pathway | Reduction in hallucinations, delusions, and hostility/aggressiveness |
| Mesocortical pathway | Increase in affective blunting, possibly other "negative" symptoms |
| Nigrostriatal pathway | Increase in extrapyramidal movements, parkinsonism, possibly tardive dyskinesia |
| Tuberoinfundibular pathway | Increase in prolactin levels, with menstrual irregularities and gynecomastia |

Aripiprazole is currently the only available partial dopamine agonist antipsychotic agent for clinical use. Its receptor binding actions are unique, in that it acts as a partial agonist at the dopamine $D_2$ and the serotonin $5\text{-}HT_{1A}$ receptors, and as an antagonist at serotonin $5\text{-}HT_{2A}$ receptors. Although its exact mechanisms of action are unclear, it is postulated that partial agonism at striatal $D_2$ receptors may prevent excessive blockade, thus explaining its low potential for EPS.

## Anticholinergics

These are adjunctive medications in the treatment of schizophrenia. They are used to counteract antipsychotic-related EPS, via what is hypothesized to be an imbalance between dopaminergic (low) and cholinergic (high) activity in the striatum.

## Antihistamines

Some of these drugs also have anticholinergic effects. An antihistamine that is sometimes used to treat EPS is diphenhydramine.

## Beta blockers

Anticholinergic agents are generally effective in treating antipsychotic-induced acute dystonia, but they perform rather poorly in the treatment of akathisia. The beta-blockers tend to be better at reducing akathisia; the exact mechanism of action is unknown. An additional potential use for the beta-blockers is to treat any hostility or aggression that is not responding to the antipsychotic medications.

## Anxiolytics

These medications can also be effective at relieving akathisia. As with the beta blockers, it is not known how the anxiolytics work to decrease akathisia, but it does not appear to be related to the reduction of anxiety. Reducing anxiety (which is common in schizophrenia) is often a goal in working with psychotic patients, and effectively treating the anxiety may limit the severity, postpone, or possibly even prevent the recurrence of psychotic decompensation.

## Mood stabilizers

There are two situations in which the addition of a mood stabilizer to an antipsychotic agent may better treat psychotic symptoms. The first is when there are significant mood symptoms coincident with the psychotic symptoms (even when criteria for schizoaffective disorder are not met). The second is in cases of clozapine-resistant psychosis. The rationale for adding the mood stabilizer is that an alternative hypothesis to the dopamine hypothesis of schizophrenia is that of the glutamate hyperfunction hypothesis. The anticonvulsant/mood stabilizer lamotrigine, which acts as a glutamate release inhibitor, has been shown to effectively augment the antipsychotic effects of clozapine, as well as other antipsychotic medications.

## Antidepressants

These medications are probably under-utilized in the treatment of schizophrenic patients, as depression is quite common in this population. Suicide is also common in schizophrenia, with depression an important risk factor; therefore, the use of antidepressant medications should be considered in patients with schizophrenia who are also experiencing more than a mild dysphoria.

## Sedative-hypnotics

Sleep disturbances are common complaints in persons with schizophrenia and other psychotic disorders. Unresolved poor sleep can fuel anxiety, irritability, agitation, and even psychosis. It can contribute to use of alcohol or illicit substances by patients as an attempt to "self-medicate" their insomnia. Agents from this class of medications may be useful, short-term adjuncts to the other medications mentioned in this section.

## Dosages

The dosage recommendations for the medications mentioned in Table 8.2 are based mostly on extrapolations from prescribing information for adults, or from limited studies involving children and adolescents. A generally safe guideline to follow states that if a dosage range for a medication is suggested, that the patient be started at the lower end of the range. Sometimes a little bit of medication can yield dramatic results; dosing can always be increased if the previous amount was ineffective, but tolerated.

## Antipsychotics

The dosage ranges for these medications are quite broad, and vary depending on relative strength. The potency of the FGAs was usually based on chlorpromazine equivalents (CPZ-E). It was felt that at least 100 mg of daily CPZ was needed to achieve antipsychotic activity. Since the SGAs have been available, and more sophisticated receptor binding studies have been completed, the concept of CPZ-E has been less useful. It has been demonstrated that there is actually a somewhat narrow therapeutic window for these medications, in that antipsychotic effects require 65–70% $D_2$ receptor occupancy by the drug, whereas 80% or greater occupancy produces EPS. As there are no good ways of measuring receptor occupancy in routine practice, dosing of antipsychotic medications remains a clinical skill.

## Anticholinergics

The listed dosages for the agents in this class should be sufficient to abort episodes of EPS. The use of prophylactic anticholinergic medications in adults is controversial; they should not be used in children and adolescents.

## Antihistamines

The dosing of diphenhydramine for relief of EPS is generally similar to doses used for the treatment of allergies. There may be situations in which higher doses will be required; the patient should be carefully watched for adverse effects (see "Side Effects" below).

## Beta-blockers (see Chapter 7)

The use of these medications is begun with fairly conservative dosages. Propranolol may be the easiest beta-blocker to use, as dosing is correlated with patient weight, i.e. 10–20 mg twice daily for < 35 kg, or 20–40 kg twice daily for > 35 kg.

## Anxiolytics (see Chapter 4)

These medications are also initiated in a cautious fashion. Acute, short-term anxiety states can be treated with short-acting agents such as lorazepam, beginning with as little as 0.25–0.5 mg every 6–8 hours. More chronic anxiety states should be treated with longer-acting agents such as clonazepam, starting with 0.25–0.5 mg every 8–12 hours.

## Mood stabilizers (see Chapter 7)

The choice of agent will determine how the medication will be dosed, i.e. whether it will be by a combination of clinical response and blood level (e.g. with lithium or valproate), or only by clinical indicators.

## Antidepressants (see Chapter 6)

Dosing of these medications is purely clinical. As there is a lag between achieving a steady-state level in the blood and clinical response, there is a temptation to prematurely increase the dose of the antidepressant. Patience is required on the part of the patient, the family, and the clinician, as adequate antidepressant doses may need up to 12 weeks to demonstrate efficacy.

## Sedative-hypnotics (see Chapter 11)

These medications should be used at the lowest effective doses possible. Overzealous efforts to help the patient may eventually cause more problems than they solve (see the following section).

## Side effects (adverse effects)

This section will address the unwanted, harmful, and/or potentially fatal effects of medications that are used in the treatment of schizophrenia. Their more common – and usually benign – side effects (e.g. headache, stomach upset, and sedation) will not be covered in detail.

### Antipsychotics

The major adverse effects of concern include:

**Table 8.4** Antipsychotic medications and risk of extrapyramidal symptoms.

| Class | Agent | Relative risk[a] |
|---|---|---|
| *First-generation* | | |
| Phenothiazines | Chlorpromazine | 2 |
| | Thioridazine | 1 |
| | Fluphenazine | 3 |
| | Perphenazine | 2–3 |
| | Trifluoperazine | 3 |
| Butyrophenones | Haloperidol | 3 |
| Miscellaneous | Loxapine | 2–3 |
| | Molindone | 1 |
| | Thiothixene | 3 |
| *Second-generation* | Clozapine | 0 |
| | Risperidone | 2 |
| | Olanzapine | 1 |
| | Quetiapine | 0 |
| | Ziprasidone | 1 |
| *Partial DA agonist* | Aripiprazole | 0–1 |

[a] On a 0 (negligible) to 3 (high) scale.

- Extrapyramidal symptoms. These are defined as *acute dystonias, pseudo-parkinsonism, akathisia,* or *tardive dyskinesia.* Dystonias are muscular spasms that usually, but not exclusively, involve the head, neck, and back. They are frightening to both patients and providers. They are considered an emergency if they cause respiratory distress or oculogyria; treatment with an anticholinergic agent is indicated (see "How to use the medications" below). Pseudo-parkinsonism can be indistinguishable from idiopathic Parkinson's disease. It can adversely affect a patient's ability to function. Akathisia is a subjective sense of restlessness and inability to relax. It is usually – but not always – associated with observable psychomotor agitation. Unresolved akathisia may be a factor in the suicides of some schizophrenic patients. The persistent involuntary movements of tardive dyskinesia (TD) tend to be more common in older patients, but can be seen at any age. Risk increases with duration of treatment; younger people with EOS and COS may be at greater risk. As TD is irreversible, preventive efforts are crucial. The FGAs as a group cause more EPS than do the SGAs or aripiprazole. Clozapine has the lowest incidence of EPS. Table 8.4 summarizes the relative risks of developing EPS from the use of antipsychotic medications.

**Table 8.5** Antipsychotic medications and risks of adverse metabolic effects.

| Class | Agent | ↑ weight[a] | ↑ glucose[a] | ↑ lipids[b] |
|---|---|---|---|---|
| First generation antipsychotics | | | | 1.26 |
| Phenothiazines | Chlorpromazine | 2 | 1 | – |
| | Thioridazine | 2 | 1 | – |
| | Fluphenazine | 0 | 1 | – |
| | Perphenazine | 1 | 1 | – |
| | Trifluoperazine | 0 | 1 | – |
| Butyrophenones | Haloperidol | 0 | 1 | – |
| Miscellaneous | Loxapine | 1 | 1 | – |
| | Molindone | 2 | 1 | – |
| | Thiothixene | 0 | 1 | – |
| Second generation antipsychotics | Clozapine | 3 | 2 | 1.82 |
| | Risperidone | 1 | 1 | 1.53 |
| | Olanzapine | 3 | 2 | 1.56 |
| | Quetiapine | 2 | 1 | 1.52 |
| | Ziprasidone | 0 | 1 | 1.40 |
| *Partial DA agonist* | Aripiprazole | 0 | 1 | 1.19 |

[a] Relative risk: scale from 0 (negligible) to 3 (high).

[b] Odds ratios[OR](based on adult data); OR reference 1.00 (no antipsychotic use).

- Neuroleptic malignant syndrome (NMS). This is a serious adverse condition which can be caused by any antipsychotic, but especially the high-potency ones (such as haloperidol). Up to one-third of patients with NMS will die, so early recognition and removal of the offending agent(s) are paramount. Symptoms include an increase in body temperature, pulse, respiratory rate, muscle tone, and diaphoresis, with an associated change in level of consciousness (see "How to monitor the medications" for laboratory studies to pursue if NMS is suspected).
- Metabolic changes. The weight gain, hyperglycemia, and/or hyperlipidemia associated with antipsychotic agents are especially problematic side effects in younger people. Adverse metabolic changes vary relative to the medications used, with the SGAs, as a group, more likely to affect metabolic parameters than do the FGAs (Table 8.5 compares individual SGAs and aripiprazole in terms of these effects).
- Endocrine changes. The primary effect in this category is hyperprolactinemia, which, as previously mentioned, is caused by

**Table 8.6** Antipsychotic medications and risk of hyperprolactinemia.

| Class | Agent | Relative risk[a] |
|---|---|---|
| *First generation antipsychotics* | | |
| Phenothiazines | Chlorpromazine | 2 |
| | Thioridazine | 2 |
| | Fluphenazine | 2 |
| | Perphenazine | 2 |
| | Trifluoperazine | 2 |
| Butyrophenones | Haloperidol | 2 |
| Miscellaneous | Loxapine | 2 |
| | Molindone | 2 |
| | Thiothixene | 2 |
| *Second generation antipsychotics* | Clozapine | 0 |
| | Risperidone | 2 |
| | Olanzapine | 1 |
| | Quetiapine | 0 |
| | Ziprasidone | 1 |
| *Partial DA agonist* | Aripiprazole | 0 |

[a] On a 0 (negligible) to 3 (high) scale.

dopamine blockade in the tuberoinfundibular pathway. Clinical signs and symptoms include galactorrhea and menstrual irregularities, including amenorrhea. Long-term elevations of prolactin may promote osteoporosis. Table 8.6 lists antipsychotic medications and their relative tendencies to increase serum prolactin.

- Agranulocytosis. The risk of developing this hematologic problem was reported infrequently during the era of FGA use. Of the newer antipsychotic medications, quetiapine has also been infrequently associated with agranulocytosis. The medication that is associated with a greater risk (slightly greater than 1% of patients over one year) is clozapine (see "How to monitor the medications" below).
- Seizures. All of the antipsychotics – older and newer – can cause seizures. They are more likely to occur at higher doses and in individuals with a higher risk of having seizures. The prescribing information for clozapine contains a specific warning in this regard.
- Myocarditis. Risperidone and ziprasidone have rarely been associated with the development of myocarditis. The rate of myocarditis in patients treated with clozapine is significantly greater than that seen in the

general population; a specific warning is included in the drug's prescribing information.

- Hypotension. Decreases in blood pressure related to changes in bodily posture (i.e. orthostatic hypotension) can occur with any antipsychotic agent. The orthostasis associated with the use of clozapine can be quite serious, including to the point of syncope, or even cardio-respiratory collapse. The prescribing information for clozapine also carries a warning for this problem.
- Other cardiac effects. Prolongation of the $QT_C$ interval (a risk factor for *torsades de pointes*) is a dose-related phenomenon that can occur during the use of either thioridazine or ziprasidone. The risk of other types of cardiac conduction abnormalities, from the routine use of antipsychotics, is relatively low. The greatest risk, however, is in the setting of antipsychotic toxicity, related to either inadvertent overdosing or an intentional suicide attempt.

## Anticholinergics

Common side effects include dry mouth, blurred vision, constipation, difficulty urinating, restlessness, or sedation. More serious effects of concern include hyperthermia, vomiting, paralytic ileus, tachycardia, and mental status changes, such as delirium. These medications are used to treat the EPS caused by antipsychotic agents, which may have their own inherent anticholinergic activity. The combined use of both types of medications may greatly increase the risk of anticholinergic toxicity.

## Antihistamines

Side effects – and cautions – are similar to those related to the anticholinergic agents.

## Beta-blockers

Common side effects include dizziness, fatigue, bradycardia, mental status changes, gastrointestinal upset, and various skin rashes. Less common – but more serious – adverse events can be bronchospasm and heart failure, both of which may occur more readily in children. Addition of these agents to medications that also increase the risk for cardiac and/or respiratory adverse effects (e.g. the antipsychotics) should be done with great caution.

## Anxiolytics

The benzodiazepines can cause sedation, behavioral disinhibition (such as seen in alcohol intoxication), cognitive impairment, and withdrawal agitation. The combination of these medications with clozapine greatly increases the risk of serious cardiac and/or respiratory dysfunction.

## Mood stabilizers

Common lithium side effects include increased thirst and urine volumes, fine hand tremors, gastrointestinal upset, and leukocytosis. More serious associated conditions include hypothyroidism, renal insufficiency, cardiac arrhythmias, diarrhea with electrolyte disturbances, and lithium toxicity.

The anticonvulsant mood stabilizers can elevate liver function tests values. They have also been associated with Stevens–Johnson syndrome and toxic epidermal necrolysis (except with gabapentin). Hepatic failure has been reported with valproic acid and carbamazepine. Lamotrigine has reportedly caused multi-organ failure. Valproic acid can cause severe pancreatitis, as well as thrombocytopenia. Aplastic anemia and agranulocytosis have been reported with carbamazepine. Gabapentin may cause a transient hyponatremia early in the course of treatment. Topiramate commonly causes impaired concentration, weight loss, paresthesias, and nephrolithiasis. Carbamazepine, oxcarbazepine, and topiramate may reduce the efficacy of oral contraceptives. The addition of any of these medications to an antipsychotic regimen increases the risk of medicine–medicine interactions and more side effects. Anticonvulsants increase risk for suicidality (FDA, 2008).

## Antidepressants

The SSRI antidepressants can cause agitation, akathisia, and hypomania, which could be misattributed to worsening of the psychosis or side effects from the antipsychotic agent. The SSRIs can cause the serotonin syndrome, especially when they are used concomitantly with other serotonergic agents, such as the SGAs. Bupropion can lower the seizure threshold (see "Contraindications" below). With the exception of bupropion and mirtazapine, all of the commonly used antidepressants can cause hyponatremia and/or SIADH. As the antipsychotics may also lower serum sodium, their combination with antidepressants increases the potential for serious hyponatremia. Nefazodone can cause hepatic failure; it is only available as a generic in the USA.

## Sedative-hypnotics

The main concern in using these agents to treat psychotic patients is the potential for synergism with other psychotropic medications, increasing the risk of oversedation and associated adverse events (e.g. falls and injuries).

# Contraindications

Unless stated otherwise, the reader should assume that any medication will have as a contraindication sensitivity to that medication or any of its constituents.

## Antipsychotics

As a group, the FGAs are contraindicated in patients with blood dyscrasias, hepatic damage, subcortical brain damage, and obtundation. The use of thioridazine is also contraindicated in patients with congenital long $QT_C$ syndrome, who are taking other medications that can prolong the $QT_C$ interval, or who already have cardiac arrhythmias.

The SGAs, as a group, do not carry any specific contraindications; there are, however, some exceptions. The cautions about potential cardiac arrhythmias during the use of ziprasidone are similar to those associated with thioridazine. Clozapine should not be used in patients with myeloproliferative disorders, poorly controlled epilepsy, paralytic ileus, previous clozapine-related adverse hematologic reactions, or concurrent use of other medications with the potential to suppress bone marrow function.

## Anticholinergics

These medications should not be used in patients with narrow angle glaucoma, as they may precipitate angle closure and increase intraocular pressure. This may be potentiated by the inherent anticholinergic activity of the antipsychotics.

## Antihistamines

Although not contraindicated, these medications should be used with extreme caution in patients with narrow angle glaucoma, stenosing peptic ulcer, or pyloroduodenal obstruction.

## Beta-blockers

These agents should not be used in patients with sinus bradycardia and greater than first-degree block, asthma, sick sinus syndrome, significant peripheral arterial disease, pheochromocytoma, and right ventricular failure associated with pulmonary hypertension.

## Anxiolytics

The benzodiazepines are contraindicated in the presence of narrow angle glaucoma. The combined use of a benzodiazepine with clozapine is relatively contraindicated.

## Mood stabilizers

Lithium should not be used in patients with severe cardiovascular disease, renal disease (without dialysis), dehydration, sodium depletion, or on medications that can lower serum sodium levels. Carbamazepine should be avoided in persons with a history of bone marrow suppression, as well as in individuals with acute intermittent porphyria. Valproic acid is contraindicated in the presence of significant hepatic dysfunction or a urea cycle disorder.

## Antidepressants

The concomitant use of thioridazine and fluoxetine (and for at least 5 weeks after discontinuation) or paroxetine is contraindicated, as the combination can elevate thioridazine levels and the $QT_c$ interval. Concurrent use of antidepressants with pimozide should be avoided, as the combination can increase the $QT_c$ interval. Bupropion is contraindicated in patients with a seizure disorder, in those with bulimia nervosa or anorexia nervosa, or in those withdrawing from CNS sedatives (including alcohol).

## Sedative-hypnotics

No specific contraindications for these agents, except for chloral hydrate, which should not be used in patients with clinically significant hepatic or renal impairment.

## How to use the medications

### Antipsychotics

Despite the lack of well-designed studies with large numbers of subjects, the use of antipsychotic medications for EOS and COS is both reasonable and compassionate. What is unclear is which type of antipsychotic to choose (i.e. FGA, SGA, or partial dopamine agonist) as the first treatment. Some researchers argue that the newer agents offer advantages over the older agents, given their lower incidence of EPS and cognitive dysfunction, better treatment of negative symptoms. Others question the efficacy of the modern agents for negative symptoms, and express concern about their metabolic and endocrine effects, especially in younger patients.

Once factors such as side effects and contraindications are taken into consideration, the agent chosen should be started at a dose sufficient to control symptoms such as hallucinations, agitation, and aggression, but not cause sedation that interferes with the ability to participate in psychological and social therapies, and educational efforts.

Most clinicians – and parents – are likely to feel more comfortable starting with an SGA. The first increase in dose can occur as early as 2 weeks after initiation, with subsequent increases at biweekly intervals until symptoms are well-controlled, side effects become bothersome, or a target dosage is reached. A medication trial should be considered adequate after a minimum of 4–6 weeks of appropriate dosing. Before considering a trial of clozapine, the patient should have failed at least two adequate trials of an FGA, an SGA, and/or a partial dopamine agonist (aripiprazole).

Some primary care physicians may consider psychiatric consultation before or after initiating treatment with clozapine; some others may consider transfer of care to a psychiatrist. In the event of clozapine-resistance in a patient, the primary care physician should seriously consider referring the patient to a psychiatrist.

### Anticholinergics

As noted previously in Table 8.4, some antipsychotic medications are more likely to cause EPS than others: the high-potency FGAs such as haloperidol, fluphenazine, and trifluoperazine; the SGAs risperidone, olanzapine, and ziprasidone. Patients at high risk for developing dystonia are males of African ancestry. The anticholinergics can be used either orally or parenterally; the former will last longer, the latter will work faster in alleviating the dystonia. These medications are minimally effective for akathisia.

## Antihistamines

Diphenhydramine can be used in a manner similar to the anticholinergic agents. It tends to be more sedating, so may be a good choice for patients with dystonia and agitation.

## Beta blockers

These agents have been used to treat the akathisia produced by the antipsychotic medications. The lipophilic beta blockers (such as propranolol and metoprolol) are more effective than the hydrophilic ones (e.g. atenolol and nadolol).

## Anxiolytics

The benzodiazepines can effectively reduce the anxiety seen in schizophrenic patients. They are a good second choice for akathisia that is not responding to the beta blockers.

## Mood stabilizers

The addition of lithium, carbamazepine, or valproate to an antipsychotic may improve treatment response, but only if there are prominent affective symptoms, i.e. the patient likely has schizoaffective disorder.

## Antidepressants

Clinically significant depression that coexists with psychosis may need to be treated with antidepressant medications, although studies to date are inconclusive regarding the efficacy of this strategy. Most of the studies involved older antidepressants. The few studies that look at SSRIs for depression in schizophrenia suggest that sertraline may be beneficial. Worsening of mood after starting an antidepressant could indicate a cyclic mood component; the antidepressant should be tapered off or discontinued. An increase of agitation could be from akathisia secondary to the SSRI; its management would be similar to that for antipsychotic-induced akathisia.

## Sedative-hypnotics

Lack of sleep can precipitate or exacerbate psychosis. It is important to help patients re-establish a healthy sleep cycle; short-term use of sedative or hypnotic agents may facilitate that process.

# How to monitor the medications (including what tests are needed)

## Antipsychotics

There are strict guidelines for the monitoring of patients on clozapine. Before starting the medication, and during the course of treatment, the patient's white blood cell (WBC) count should be $\geq 3500/mm^2$ and the absolute neutrophil count (ANC) should be $\geq 2000/mm^2$. The WBC and ANC are checked weekly for the first 6 months of treatment, every 2 weeks for months 6–12, and every 4 weeks thereafter, provided that values remain at or above the established cutoffs (detailed prescribing information is available from the manufacturers). When considering the use of clozapine, a baseline EEG should be obtained in anyone suspected of having, or at risk for, a seizure disorder. Blood pressure and pulse should be checked routinely during treatment with clozapine, especially during initiation and dosage increases. Any symptoms referable to the cardiovascular system warrant an appropriate medical evaluation.

It is important that the patient's height, weight, and BMI be measured before starting antipsychotic medications and at each subsequent visit. Blood pressure and pulse should be checked at baseline, and then no less often than every 3 months. Fasting glucose and lipids should be measured before starting treatment, 3 months afterwards, and then every 6 months thereafter. A baseline examination for abnormal neuromotor (extrapyramidal) signs is suggested, with re-checks during dosage escalations, and, once stable, every 3 months. The only atypical antipsychotic that requires baseline and follow-up ECGs is ziprasidone, particularly during dosage titrations. Prolactin should be checked at any point if menstrual abnormalities or sexual problems (in either sex) are present.

## Anticholinergics

Check blood pressure, pulse, and temperature for any elevations that could signify toxicity.

## Antihistamines

No routine laboratory tests are recommended for this class of medications.

## Beta-blockers

Blood pressure and pulse should be routinely monitored. Propranolol can occasionally elevate serum potassium, AST, ALT, and alkaline phosphatase in hypertensive patients. Pindolol may also occasionally elevate AST, ALT, alkaline phosphatase, LDH and uric acid.

## Anxiolytics

During long-term treatment with a benzodiazepine, periodic blood testing of the WBC (to check for neutropenia) and liver function tests (to check for hyperbilirubinemia or elevated LDH) is recommended.

## Mood stabilizers

Before starting lithium obtain baseline electrolytes, BUN, creatinine, thyroid function tests, WBC, and urine specific gravity; repeat 1 or 2 times/year, once the patient is stabilized. A serum lithium trough level (10–12 hours after last dose) should be measured 4–5 days after starting the medication, 4–5 days after any dosage increase, and every 3–6 months during the maintenance phase.

In patients on valproic acid or carbamazepine, baseline and follow-up (every 6–12 months) AST, ALT, LDH, and CBC should be measured. The drug level should be checked 1–2 weeks after initiation or after each dosage increase, and also every 3–6 months during maintenance. The other agents in this class do not require routine laboratory testing.

## Antidepressants

No routine laboratory tests are required for any of these medications. Venlafaxine, however, may raise serum cholesterol, so checking levels should be considered during extended treatment. The selegiline patch may elevate liver function test values, but routine testing is not necessary.

## Sedative-hypnotics

No routine laboratory tests are recommended for this class of medications.

# ■ Summary

The treatment of patients with EOS and COS may be delayed, due to limited information regarding efficacy of the antipsychotics in those populations, confusion regarding the FGA vs. SGA choice, and concerns about medication side effects. Once the commitment to treat has been made, there are three basic options: the use of an FGA, the use of an SGA, or the use of an PDAA (partial dopamine agonist). Figure 8.1 is a guide to the treatment sequence to follow, no matter which type of antipsychotic agent is chosen first. If adequate trials are not effective at Level I and Level II, a choice needs to made between one more trial of a standard antipsychotic medication (Level IIIA) or clozapine (Level IIIB), the ultimate single-agent option. Nonresponse at Level IIIB dictates specialty referral and care.

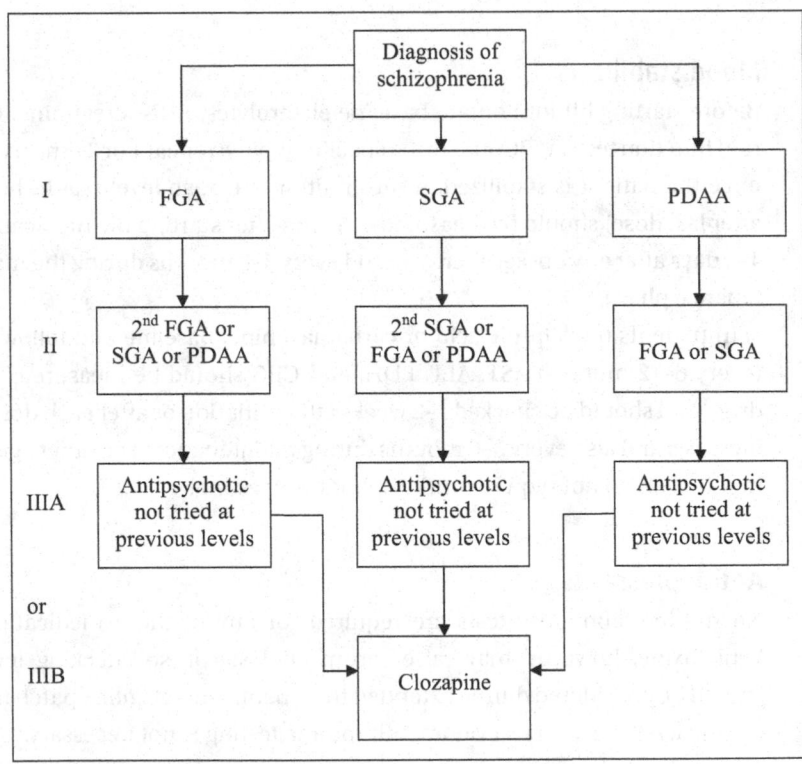

**Figure 8.1** Algorithm for treatment of early-onset schizophrenia (EOS) and childhood-onset schizophrenia (COS). FGA, First-generation antipsychotic; SGA, Second-generation antipsychotic; PDAA, Partial dopamine agonist.

Armenteros JL, Davies M. 2006. Antipsychotics in early onset schizophrenia: systematic review and meta-analysis. *Eur. Child Adolesc. Psychiatry*, 15(3):141–8.

Asarnow JR, Tompson MC, McGrath EP. 2004. Annotation: childhood-onset schizophrenia: clinical and treatment issues. *J. Child Psychol. Psychiatry*, 45(2): 180–94.

Correll CU, Penzner JB, Parikh UH *et al.* 2006. Recognizing and monitoring adverse events of second-generation antipsychotics in children and adolescents. *Child Adolesc. Psychiatric Clin. N. Am.*, 15:177–206.

Gardner DM, Baldessarini RJ, Waraich P. 2005. Modern antipsychotic drugs: a critical overview. *Can. Med. Assoc. J.*, 172(13):1703–11.

Gonthier M, Lyon MA. 2004. Childhood-onset schizophrenia: an overview. *Psychol. Schools*, 41(7):803–11.

Robinson DG, Woerner MG, Delman HM, Kane JM. 2005. Pharmacological treatments for first-episode schizophrenia. *Schizophr. Bull.*, 31(3):705–22. Epub 2005 Jul 8.

Ropcke B, Eggers C. 2005. Early-onset schizophrenia. *Eur. Child Adolesc. Psychiatry*, 14(6):341–50.

www.fda.gov/medwatch/safety/2008/safety08.htm#Antiepileptic

# Autism spectrum disorders

## 9

## ■ Definition

Autism spectrum disorders (ASD) are characterized by deficits in social interaction, verbal and nonverbal communication and repetitive, stereotypical behaviors and interests. These impairments are severe, pervasive and deviant relative to the child's developmental level and mental age. Each child will display a wide range of individual variability in the behavioral symptoms. Most children manifest the early symptoms and are diagnosed between ages 18 months and 36 months; in many, diagnosis can be suspected as early as 10–12 months of age and in most by 24 months. Autism should be suspected when an infant does not babble, point, or make meaningful gestures by 1 year of age; does not speak one word by 16 months; does not combine two words by 2 years of age; does not respond to name; and loses language or social skills. Autistic disorder is classified as one of the pervasive developmental disorders according to the DSM–IV–TR; the others are Rett's disorder, childhood disintegrative disorder, Asperger's disorder, and pervasive developmental disorder not otherwise specified.

## ■ Epidemiology

Over the past several years there has been an increase in reported prevalence of ASD, and it is currently estimated to range from 2–6 per 1000 children. The reasons for the increase in the incidence of reported cases of autism are not clear and it is generally recognized that a combination of factors including increased awareness, broader definition, improved diagnosis, or a true increase in autism have been implicated. Autism has been reported to be 2–4 times more common in males than in females.

# ■ Differential diagnoses/comorbidity

Autistic disorder should be distinguished from other pervasive developmental disorders; the differential includes:

- Autistic disorder. This is generally recognized by 3 years of age, and is associated with significant impairment in social skills. The cognitive abilities of children with autistic disorder can range from normal to severe mental retardation (MR).
- Asperger's disorder. This is typically recognized after 4 years of age. Children with Asperger's disorder also have significant deficits in social skills, but their communication skills may be only mildly affected, and their IQ range from normal to mild MR.
- Rett's disorder and childhood disintegrative disorder. In both there is a loss or regression of previously acquired developmental skills.
  - In Rett's disorder there is deceleration of head growth and it is typically recognized by 2 years of age.
  - Children with childhood disintegrative disorder generally present after 2 years of age with loss of skills, severe deficits in communication skills, and severe MR.
- Pervasive developmental disorder not otherwise specified (PDD-NOS). This term is used for those children who have impaired social skills and a variable degree of other autistic features, but do not meet specific criteria for any of the other diagnoses.
- Childhood schizophrenia. This has a later onset (usually in adolescence, rarely before puberty) and is associated with hallucinations and delusions.
- Specific language impairment. Children with these disorders have normal social development and normal intelligence.
- Mental retardation. Children with MR have deficits in cognitive abilities and their social and emotional development is commensurate with their mental age. The social development in children with MR though delayed is not deviant.

# ■ Pharmacotherapy

The classification, mechanisms of action, side effects, contraindications, and monitoring guidelines of various medications used in children and adolescents with autism are described in detail in other chapters. The following comments relate to their use specifically in children with autism.

## Antipsychotic agents

Risperidone is approved by the US FDA for use in children and adolescents (age 5 years and above) with autistic disorder. It is indicated for the treatment of the symptoms of irritability that include aggression, deliberate self-injury, and temper tantrums associated with autistic disorder. The dosage of risperidone should be individualized based on the clinical response and tolerability. Dosing should be initiated at 0.25 mg per day for children less than 20 kg of body weight, and at 0.5 mg per day for those who weigh 20 kg or more. The total daily oral dose can be given once daily or can be divided into twice daily regimen. After a minimum of 4 days from the initiation of the treatment the dose may be increased to the recommended daily dose of 0.5 mg for children who weigh less than 20 kg and to 1 mg for those who weigh 20 kg or more. The recommended dose should be maintained for 2 weeks to assess the clinical response. In children whose response is judged to be inadequate an increase in the daily dose may be considered at about 2-week intervals in the increments of 0.25 mg per day for children who weigh less than 20 mg and 0.5 mg per day for those 20 kg or more. Typical dosage to which clinical response has been reported is between 0.5 mg and 2.5 mg per day. Sedation, weight gain, fatigue, and constipation are the most common side effects reported. A once-daily dose at bedtime or total dose divided twice daily or reduction in total daily dose may help reduce the sedation during the daytime. Hyperprolactinemia is also a significant side effect in adolescents.

Other atypical antipsychotic agents have been less well studied and data are insufficient at this time to make any judgement about their safety or efficacy in children and adolescents with ASD.

## Antidepressant agents

Use of selective serotonin reuptake inhibitors (SSRIs) is common in children and adolescents with ASD. Although some of the SSRIs have been approved for use in children and adolescents with depression and

**Table 9.1** Typical dosages of selective serotonin reuptake inhibitors.

| Agent | Daily dosage range |
| --- | --- |
| Citalopram | 5–40 mg |
| Escitalopram | 5–20 mg |
| Fluvoxamine | 12.5–300 mg |
| Fluoxetine | 5–60 mg |
| Paroxetine | 5–40 mg |
| Sertraline | 12.5–200 mg |

obsessive-compulsive disorders, none is approved by the FDA for use in the symptomatic treatment of children and adolescents with ASD. As a class, these agents have been reported to be beneficial in reducing anxiety symptoms, obsessions, compulsive behaviors, repetitive stereotypical behaviors, and improving mood. Short-term safety and efficacy based on controlled trials have been reported for fluoxetine and fluvoxamine, and there is reason to believe that ongoing trials of other SSRIs may show similar safety and efficacy profiles. The dosages for SSRIs in children and adolescents with ASD have not been established but it is recommended to start at the lowest end of the typical range (Table 9.1) and titrating the dose very slowly up to achieve desired symptomatic improvement. Availability of liquid formulations of some of the SSRIs allows for easier administration of lower dosages. It appears that children and adolescents with ASD are more likely to manifest adverse effects with the use of SSRIs and lower dosages are therefore recommended.

Clomipramine and mirtazepine have also been used in autism, for mood and anxiety symptoms, obsessions, compulsions, and repetitive behaviors. Clomipramine is a tricyclic antidepressant (TCA) with a side effect profile similar to other TCAs. It is approved by the FDA for use in children age 10 years and over for obsessive-compulsive disorder. In children the usual recommended dose is 3 mg/kg/day. In adolescents the dosages range from 100–250 mg per day.

Mirtazepine has been shown to improve target symptoms of aggression, self-injurious behaviors, hyperactivity, anxiety, depression, and sleep disturbances in adolescents and young adults. The typical daily dose of mirtazepine ranges from 7.5–45 mg. It has no FDA approved indication for use in children and adolescents (less than 18 years of age).

## Stimulant agents

Methylphenidate has been shown to be effective in improving symptoms of hyperactivity, impulsivity and inattention in children and adolescents with ASD. Compared with children who do not have ASD, children with ASD are more likely to experience side effects at usual dosages of methylphenidate, hence a very low starting dose and the lowest effective maintenance dose is recommended. Many formulations of methylphenidate are available with variable duration of action that range from 4 hours to 10 hours. Use of short to intermediate acting formulations may allow for a lower starting dose and better ability to titrate the dose. Initial dose is typically 5 mg, with increments of 2.5–5 mg weekly until effective dose is reached or intolerable side effects have been noted. The typical daily dose ranges from 5–60 mg.

## Alpha$_2$ adrenergic agonists

Both clonidine and guanfacine have been shown to be beneficial in reducing emotional outbursts, increasing frustration tolerance, decreasing startle response, improving attention, and some improvement in sleep. The dosages used for clonidine are 5 microgram/kg/day for the transdermal patch and from 0.1 mg to 0.2 mg/day for oral administration. The dosage for guanfacine is generally from 0.5 mg to 2 mg per dose given orally up to three times daily.

## ■ Summary

The mainstay of treatment of children and adolescents with autism spectrum disorders is an appropriate individualized education program and behavioral therapy. Many treatment models for educational and behavioral therapy have been described. Pharmacological treatment is not the primary treatment for autism, and no medications have been shown to improve the core symptoms of impaired social relatedness and impaired communication, either verbal or nonverbal. Use of specific medication is considered for specific target symptom or symptoms cluster (Table 9.2). Target symptoms must be clearly identified and documented so that effects of the medication can be assessed. Use of medications often allows for more effective participation by children in educational and behavioral treatments

**Table 9.2** Target symptoms and medications.

| Target symptom or symptom cluster | Pharmacological agents used |
| --- | --- |
| Irritability, aggression, self-injurious behaviors, temper tantrums | • Risperidone<br>• Data limited for other atypical antipsychotic agents |
| Mood changes, anxiety, obsessions, compulsions, repetitive, and stereotypical behaviors | • SSRIs have been shown to ameliorate symptoms to a variable degree<br>• Other agents used are clomipramine and mirtazepine |
| Hyperactivity, impulsivity, inattention | • Methylphenidate has been shown to be effective at low dosages<br>• Other agents with variable efficacy clonidine and guanfacine |

by controlling interfering behaviors. Children with autism are more pre-disposed to the side effects of pharmacological agents, and a low starting dose and a slow increase is recommended to achieve the lowest effective dosage.

## SELECTED BIBLIOGRAPHY

American Academy of Child and Adolescent Psychiatry. 2007. *Practice Parameter: Pervasive Developmental Disorders.* www.aacap.org

American Academy of Pediatrics. 2007. *Autism: Caring for Children with Autism Spectrum Disorders: A Resource Toolkit for Clinicians.* Elk Grove Village, IL: American Academy of Pediatrics.

American Medical Association. 2007. Special issue on autism. *Archives of Pediatrics and Adolescent Medicine*, 161(4):313–424.

American Psychiatric Association. 2000. *Diagnostic and Statistical Manual of Mental Disorders, Fourth edition, Text Revision.* Washington DC: APA, pp. 69–84.

Barbaresi WJ, Katusic SK, Voigt RG. 2006. Autism: a review of the state of the art science for pediatric primary health care clinicians, *Arch. Pediatr. Adolesc. Med.*, 160:1167–75.

Carr JE, LeBlanc LA. 2007. Autism spectrum disorders. *Primary Care Clinics in Office Practice*, 36(2):343–59.

Huff MB, Deokar AM, Omar H. 2008. Autism spectrum disorders in adolescents: psychosocial aspects and management. *Pediatric. Clin. N. Am.*, 55: in press.

Johnson CP, Myers S, and the Council on Children with Disabilities. 2007. Identification and evaluation of children with autism spectrum disorders. *Pediatrics*, 120:1183–215.

King BH, Bostic JQ. 2006. An update on pharmacologic treatments for autism spectrum disorders. *Child Adolesc. Psychiatr. Clin. N. Am.*, 15:161–75.

Kolevzon A, Gross R, Reichenberg A. 2007. Prenatal and perinatal risk factors for autism: a review and integration of findings. *Arch. Pediatr. Adolesc. Med.*, 161:326–33.

McCracken JT, McGough J, Shah B *et al.* 2002. Risperidone in children with autism and serious behavioral problems. *N. Engl. J Med.*, 347(5):314–21.

Myers S and the Council on Children with Disabilities. 2007. Management of children with autism. *Pediatrics*, 120:1162–82.

Posey DJ, Erickson CA, Stigler KA, McDougle CJ. 2006. The use of selective serotonin reuptake inhibitors in autism and related disorders. *J. Child Adolesc. Psychopharmacol.*, 16(1/2):181–6.

Rapin I, Tuchman R. 2008. Autism: definition, neurobiology, screening, and diagnosis. *Pediatr. Clin. N. Am.*, 55: in press.

Schonfeld DJ, Manning-Courtney P. 2007. Looking ahead to even more discoveries in autism spectrum disorder while addressing current needs. *Arch. Pediatr.*, 161:412–13.

Volkmar FR, Pauls D. 2003. Autism. *Lancet*, 362:1133–41.

## 10

# Psychotropic management of children and adolescents with cognitive–adaptive disabilities

The presence of cognitive impairments – either congenital or acquired – can have profound effects on a child or adolescent's development. They place him or her at higher risk for behavioral and psychiatric disorders. Those same disturbances can also place a high burden of demand on families, schools, the medical system, and governmental agencies.

The purpose of this chapter is to address the cognitive, affective, and behavioral issues that these patients will present within the clinical setting, and to discuss the psychopharmacologic treatment options available to the practicing pediatrician.

## ■ Definition

The diagnosis of mental retardation requires that the individual in question has demonstrated a below-average intellectual quotient (IQ) on a standardized intelligence test, as well as levels of adaptive functioning that are below those expected for his or her age or culture. Commonly affected areas of functioning include communication, socialization, self-care, safety, and education.

**Table 10.1** Mental retardation (MR).

| Level of severity | IQ level |
| --- | --- |
| Mild MR | 50–55 to approximately 70 |
| Moderate MR | 35–40 to 50–55 |
| Severe MR | 20–25 to 35–40 |
| Profound MR | Below 20 or 25 |

The level of mental retardation is commonly defined by IQ score. In the DSM–IV–TR, there are four degrees of severity (Table 10.1).

# ■ Epidemiology

In the USA, the prevalence of mental retardation is somewhere between 1 and 3 out of every 100 people. In special educational settings, about 1 out of 10 students receiving services has some degree of mental retardation.

Fortunately, the majority of people with mental retardation function in the mild MR range; however, in the majority of those cases no specific etiology can be identified. Conversely, in the minority of people with severe and profound MR, the etiology is usually discovered fairly easily.

The particular cause of any one person's mental retardation may have relevance to his or her risk of psychopathology and/or medical conditions that in themselves raise the risk for psychiatric and behavioral problems. For example, when compared with the general population, those patients with Down syndrome have higher rates of maladaptive, externalizing behaviors in childhood, and depression, seizure disorders, and Alzheimer's disease as they age.

Another example is patients with Fragile X syndrome. Males with this disorder are at greater risk of developing seizures and autism. About 4 out of 5 males with Fragile X syndrome have symptoms consistent with Attention-deficit/hyperactivity disorder (ADHD), and approximately 1 out of 3 girls will also show ADHD symptoms. The risk for depression in Fragile X females increases with age, and is greater than the rate seen in females without the disorder.

Lastly, even though most individuals with Fetal alcohol syndrome have IQs in the normal range, some may be as low as the severe MR level. In those with higher intellectual functioning, there is still a greater risk for

ADHD symptoms, learning disorders, substance-use disorders (especially alcohol abuse and dependence), depression, psychosis, and sociopathy.

Down syndrome, Fragile X syndrome, and Fetal alcohol syndrome are the most common, identifiable causes of mental retardation. The combined number of people with those disorders, however, accounts for only about 30% of the total cases of mental retardation.

# Differential diagnosis/comorbidity

The evaluation of a patient with intellectual impairment should be carried out in a careful and thoughtful manner, and is required before any sort of pharmacologic intervention is to be instituted. The three diagnostic domains to consider are: (1) the cause (etiology) of the mental retardation; (2) conditions that can mimic mental retardation; and (3) conditions that can be comorbid with the mental retardation. Tables 10.2, 10.3 and 10.4 list the more common disorders in each domain.

# Psychopharmacology

Individuals with intellectual impairment, as previously noted, can present with a myriad of emotional and behavioral signs and symptoms. It is therefore not surprising when a patient with mental retardation presents with an extensive medication history, which can include drugs from several psychotropic – and nonpsychotropic – classes.

Given that we are discussing the treatment of patients who are quite vulnerable, some general points regarding the pharmacotherapy of individuals with mental retardation are in order, prior to describing specific medications and indications. Firstly, mental retardation should not be thought of as an illness, but as the end result of aberrant neuronal development. As there are numerous possible causes of mental retardation, and as there are usually no specific treatments for those causal conditions, there is no specific treatment for the intellectual impairment itself. Secondly, it is usually not the intellectual deficits themselves that are the focus of medical attention, but the associated affective, cognitive, and behavioral disturbances that lead to consideration of psychopharmacologic interventions. Thirdly, as comorbidity tends to be quite common, there is an increased tendency for patients with mental retardation to be treated with multiple medications. Fourthly, people with mental retardation have brains that are sensitive

**Table 10.2** Causes of mental retardation.

| | |
|---|---|
| Chromosomal/genetic | Down syndrome |
| | Fragile X syndrome |
| | Klinefelters syndrome |
| | Lesch–Nyhan syndrome |
| | Rett's disorder |
| | Williams syndrome |
| | Prader–Willi syndrome |
| | Angelman syndrome |
| | Cri-du-chat syndrome |
| | X-linked adrenoleukodystrophy |
| | Metachromatic leukodystrophy |
| | Rubinstein–Taybi syndrome |
| | Cornelia de Lange syndrome |
| | Smith–Lemli–Opitz syndrome |
| | Smith–Magenis syndrome |
| | Tuberous sclerosis |
| | Neurofibromatosis type 1 |
| | Various mucopolysaccharidoses |
| | Phenylketonuria[a] |
| | Homocystinuria[a] |
| | Galactosemia[a] |
| | Congenital hypothyroidism[a] |
| Gestational factors | Maternal malnutrition |
| | Fetal exposure to medications (isotretinoin, cancer chemotherapy, phenytoin, valproate, warfarin) |
| | Fetal exposure to toxins (alcohol, heavy metals) |
| | Fetal exposure to infectious agents ("TORCHS," HIV, listeriosis) |
| | Aberrant neural development (spina bifida, myelomeningocele, schizencephaly, microcephaly, hydrocephalus) |
| Perinatal factors | Hypoxia/anoxia |
| | Severe prematurity |
| | Intracerebral hemorrhage/birth trauma |
| | Hyperbilirubinemia |
| | Sepsis |
| Postnatal factors | Meningitis/encephalitis |
| | Cerebral trauma |
| | Toxins (heavy metals) |
| | Infant malnutrition |
| | Severe emotional abuse/neglect |
| | Brain tumors and their treatments |

[a] Intellectual impairment can be minimized or prevented by early intervention.

**Table 10.3** Conditions that can mimic mental retardation.

Expressive language disorder
Mixed receptive-expressive language disorder
Phonological disorder
Borderline intellectual functioning (IQ 71–84)
Pervasive developmental disorders
Dementia
Schizophrenia
Sensory impairments

**Table 10.4** DSM–IV–TR Conditions comorbid with mental retardation.

| | |
|---|---|
| **Pervasive developmental disorders** | Autistic disorder |
| **Disruptive behavior disorders** | Attention deficit/hyperactivity disorder |
| | Oppositional defiant disorder |
| | Conduct disorder |
| **Feeding and eating disorders** | Pica |
| | Rumination disorder |
| | Anorexia nervosa |
| | Bulimia nervosa |
| **Tic disorders** | Tourette's disorder |
| | Stereotypic movement disorder |
| **Elimination disorders** | Encopresis |
| | Enuresis |
| **Psychotic disorders** | Schizophrenia |
| | Brief psychotic disorder |
| **Mood disorders** | Major depression |
| | Dysthymic disorder |
| | Bipolar disorder |
| **Anxiety disorders** | Agoraphobia |
| | Obsessive-compulsive disorder |
| | Social anxiety disorder |
| | Post-traumatic stress disorder |
| **Somatoform disorders** | Somatization disorder |
| | Pain disorder |
| **Sleep disorders** | Insomnia or Hypersomnia |
| | Breathing-related (apnea) sleep disorder |
| **Impulse control disorders** | Intermittent explosive disorder |
| | Kleptomania |
| | Pyromania |
| | Trichotillomania |

to the effects of medication, such that the use of polypharmacy sets them up for more medication interactions and adverse reactions. Lastly, given the inherent difficulties with communication that patients with mental retardation experience, there is a greater chance that unpleasant and intolerable medication effects will not be disclosed to the prescribing clinician; this will be discussed in more detail in the section "How to monitor medication."

Table 10.5 lists the pharmacologic classes and agents which may be used in the mentally retarded population. Recommendations for use in specific problem areas will be described in the section "How to use the medications."

## Medication classification and mechanism of action (see Table 3.1 in Chapter 3)

### Psychostimulants

The most commonly used compounds in this category are the amphetamines and methylphenidate. Amphetamines are available as dextroamphetamine sulfate (the dextro isomer of *d,l* amphetamine sulfate) or as mixed amphetamine salts (MAS), 1/4 of which is dextroamphetamine sulfate. They are non-catecholamine, sympathomimetic amines that act as stimulants in the CNS. The mechanism of action is believed to involve both reuptake blockade of dopamine and norepinephrine into the presynaptic neuron and increased release of those neurotransmitters into the synaptic cleft. Methylphenidate acts as a sympathomimetic agent, with mild CNS stimulant properties. Its putative mechanism of action is through activation of brain stem and cortical arousal systems.

A newer agent in this category is modafinil, which acts in many ways like the sympathomimetic agents, yet is unique, in that it does not bind to catecholamine receptors nor increase adrenergic activity. Its exact mechanism of promoting alertness and wakefulness is unknown.

### Antidepressants

The precise mechanisms through which these agents exert their clinical effects are unknown. The presumed common factor in their efficacy is an increase of available catecholamine neurotransmitters in the CNS, with the final – and therapeutic – result being downregulation of postsynaptic neurons. The MAO inhibitors (MAOI), as the name implies, prevent the breakdown of the monoamine neurotransmitters present in the terminal portion of presynaptic neurons. The tricyclic antidepressants

**Table 10.5** Medications used in persons with mental retardation, and ages at which use may be appropriate.[a]

| Class | Agent | Doses[a] | Ages[b] |
|---|---|---|---|
| **Psychostimulants: See Chapter 5 for details** | | | |
| **Antidepressants: See Chapter 6 for details** | | | |
| **Antipsychotics: See Chapter 8 for details** | | | |
| **Mood stabilizers** | | | |
| Lithium salts | Lithium carbonate | 25–35 mg/kg/d, div. 2–3 × /d (adj. to level) | ≥12 |
| Anticonvulsants | Carbamazepine | 7 mg/kg/d, 2–3 × /d (adj. to level) | Any (?) |
| | Valproic acid | 20 mg/kg/d, 2–3 × /d (adj. to level) | ≥10 |
| | Lamotrigine | 12.5–25 mg/d, titrated by 25 mg q 1–2 wks | ≥2 |
| | Oxcarbazepine | **20–29 kg:** 900 mg/d  **30–39 kg:** 1200 mg/d  **>39 kg:** 1800 mg/d | ≥18 |
| | Gabapentin | 100 mg, 2–3 × /d | Any (?) |
| | Topiramate | 1–3 mg/kg/d (1st wk.) 5–9 mg/kg/d, 2 × /d | ≥2 |
| **Alpha-agonists: See Chapter 5 for details** | | | |
| **Beta-blockers** | Propranolol | **<35 kg:** 10–20 mg; **>35 kg:** 20–40 mg, both at 2 × /d dosing | ≥18 (all) |
| | Metoprolol | 12.5–25 mg, 2 × /d[c] | |
| | Pindolol | 6.25–12.5 mg, 2 × /d[c] | |
| | Nadolol | 5–10 mg, 1 × /d[b] | |
| **Anxiolytics: See Chapter 4 for details** | | | |
| **Sedative-hypnotics: See Chapter 11 for details** | | | |
| **Antihistamines** | Cyproheptadine | **2–6 yr:** 2 mg, 2–3 × /d (max 12 mg/d) **7–14 yr:** 4 mg, 2–3 × /d (max 16 mg/d) **>14 yr:** max 32 mg/d | ≥2 |
| **Opioid antagonists** | Naltrexone | 0.5–2.0 mg/kg/d | ≥18 |

[a] Dosing is clinically based, unless stated otherwise.

[b] Ages (years) are for FDA-approved indications (see Table 3.1, Chapter 3, for details); use for other indications and/or at other ages is based on clinical judgement.

[c] Amounts are estimates, extrapolated from adult dosing.

OTC, Over-the-counter (nonprescription).

block reuptake, to varying degrees, of all the neurotransmitters into the presynaptic neurons. The SSRIs, also as the name implies, selectively block the reuptake of serotonin into presynaptic neurons. Antidepressants in other categories exert their effects through reuptake inhibition, pre- and/or postsynaptic antagonism, or possibly all of them.

## Antipsychotics

The exact mechanisms of action, in the treatment of psychosis, for this class of medications are unknown. A hypothesized explanation is related to their ability to antagonize dopamine receptors, and, in the case of the "atypical" or second-generation antipsychotics (SGAs), possibly also to additional serotonin receptor antagonism.

## Mood stabilizers

This class of medications is comprised of lithium salts and anticonvulsants. Lithium affects neuronal sodium transport, which may affect how nerve cells process catecholamines; however, the connection to its antimanic activity has not been adequately explained. The anticonvulsants, although they all share similar therapeutic effects, may have different mechanisms by which they exert those effects. Proposed theories include neuronal membrane stabilization, the inhibition of excitatory amino acids (such as glutamate and aspartate), and the increase of gamma amino-butyric acid (GABA), a known inhibitory neurotransmitter.

## Alpha-agonists

These agents stimulate brainstem $alpha_2$-adrenoreceptors, which effectively reduces CNS sympathetic outflow. As the sympathetic nervous system is involved in the "fight or flight" response, the alpha-agonists may serve to blunt anxiety or aggression in certain individuals.

## Beta-blockers

These agents block beta-adrenergic receptors, effectively reducing sympathetic nervous system activity. It is not known how they exert their effects in the CNS, as agents vary by degree of selectivity for $beta_1$ (mostly cardiac) and $beta_2$ (noncardiac) receptors, and also vary in degree of lipophilicity.

## Anxiolytics

The benzodiazepines in this class bind to specific receptors in the CNS, especially in the limbic system and other deep-brain structures. That binding leads to the calming effect that these medications are known for. Buspirone is a nonbenzodiazepine anxiolytic which may produce its calming effects through 5-HT$_{1A}$ receptor binding.

## Sedative-hypnotics

Most of the agents in this class are derived from benzodiazepines, and are generally avoided in patients with developmental disabilities (see "Side Effects" below). The nonbenzodiazepine hypnotic chloral hydrate seems to directly affect cortical functioning as its mechanism of action, although the specific physiology is unknown.

## Antihistamines

The agent in this class that is useful psychopharmacologically is cyproheptadine, which competes for binding at histaminergic receptors, but more importantly is a 5-HT$_{2A}$ antagonist.

## Opioid antagonists

Naltrexone is an oral opioid antagonist that is used to reduce use of alcohol and opiates. Its use in persons with developmental disabilities has been based on its presumed ability to block the effects of endogenous opiates, ending the "addiction" cycle of conditioned feedback, i.e. stopping the behavior by diminishing or eliminating the pleasure derived from it.

## Dosages (see Table 10.5)

### Psychostimulants (see also Chapter 5)

Methylphenidate has been the stimulant medication most often studied in the mentally retarded patient population. Dosing of methylphenidate has been quite variable, ranging from 0.15 mg/kg to 0.7 mg/kg per dose. Regarding the use of dextroamphetamine, the reported dosing has been in the range of 0.08–0.3 mg/kg/dose. No specific dosing-per-weight recommendations for the mixed amphetamines are available; the manufacturer suggests dosing based on age of the patient.

### Antidepressants (see also Chapter 6)

For fluoxetine, the daily dosing range is roughly 0.15–0.5 mg/kg. For the other antidepressants there are no similar dosage-weight guidelines available, so their use should follow sound clinical principles (see Chapter 3).

### Antipsychotics (see also Chapter 8)

Risperidone has been the most studied antipsychotic medication in the mentally retarded population. One dosing strategy, in children and adolescents, would be to start with no greater than 0.25 mg daily if ≤ 10 years of age, and no greater than 1–2 mg daily if older than 10 years of age. The dosing of the other second-generation antipsychotics, in younger patients, would be similar to that recommended for adults. The use of clozapine in this population, however, requires its own special considerations (see "How to use the medications" below).

### Mood stabilizers (see Table 10.5)

There are four agents from this class that can be initiated based on a dose-per-weight basis: lithium, carbamazepine, valproic acid, and topiramate. Oxcarbazepine dosing is based on weight ranges. The others are based on low-end adult dosing recommendations.

### Alpha-agonists (see also Chapter 5)

Despite their widespread use in persons with intellectual disabilities, clonidine has not been well-studied in that population, guanfacine even less so. Clonidine doses generally range from 0.025–0.3 mg daily (or no greater than 5 μg/kg daily), with most or all of the medication administered at night-time.

### Beta-blockers (see Table 10.5)

In using these medications for psychiatric disorders in the mentally retarded population, there is little in the literature to inform dosing, especially as related to children and adolescents. The dosage ranges in the table are conservative estimates which err on the side of safety.

### Anxiolytics (see also Chapter 4)

No specific dosing recommendations are available for the use of benzodiazepines in the mentally retarded population. In fact, their use is felt to be relatively contraindicated in persons with intellectual impairment. If used at all, doses should be quite low, and duration of treatment should be as brief as possible.

## Sedative-hypnotics (see also Chapter 11)

Similar dosing precautions as for the anxiolytics.

## Antihistamines (see Table 10.5)

The agent from this class that is used for purposes other than treatment of allergies is cyproheptadine. Dosing is based on the age of the patient.

## Opioid antagonists

In adults, the daily dose of naltrexone is 50 mg for the approved indications. In younger patients with developmental disorders, dosing is started low (0.5 mg/kg/day). There is no consistent titration schedule reported, but waiting at least 2 weeks in between dose increases is reasonable. The maximum recommended dose is 2 mg/kg/day.

## Side-effects (adverse effects)

### Psychostimulants (see also Chapter 5)

Persons with mental retardation may be at higher risk of stimulant-induced side effects. Observed reactions include diminished facial expressiveness, social interactions, and level of consciousness, or increased irritability, psychomotor activity (including tics), and anxiety. Insomnia may be provoked or exacerbated by stimulant use. In patients with poor dietary intake, stimulants may further reduce appetite and body weight. In patients with short stature or slow axial growth, stimulants (especially at higher doses over longer terms) may prohibit them from achieving their full growth potential.

## Antidepressants (see also Chapter 6)

The SSRI antidepressants can cause agitation, akathisia, and hypomania (which those with developmental disabilities may be at higher risk for). Another concern with the SSRIs is the serotonin syndrome, especially when they are used concomitantly with other serotonergic agents. Bupropion can lower the seizure threshold (see "Contraindications" below). With the exception of bupropion and mirtazapine, all of the commonly used antidepressants can cause hyponatremia and/or SIADH.

## Antipsychotics (see also Chapter 8)

Adverse effects from these agents include hyperglycemia, hyperlipidemia, hyperprolactinemia, extrapyramidal symptoms (EPS), and weight gain. Patients with mental retardation may be at higher risk for these side effects. As treatment with antipsychotics tends to be long-term in this population, the possible development of tardive dyskinesia is an especial concern.

The use of clozapine reduces the risk of the aforementioned side effects; however, its use places patients at risk for some serious adverse events, such as agranulocytosis, seizures, myocarditis, and orthostatic hypotension.

## Mood stabilizers

Common lithium side effects include increased thirst, polyuria, fine resting hand tremors, mild gastrointestinal upset, and leukocytosis. More serious associated conditions include hypothyroidism, renal insufficiency, cardiac arrhythmias, diarrhea with electrolyte disturbances, and lithium toxicity (with varied neurologic signs and symptoms).

All of the anticonvulsants used as mood stabilizers can elevate liver function tests values. They have also been associated with Stevens–Johnson syndrome and (except for gabapentin) toxic epidermal necrolyis. Hepatic failure has been reported with valproic acid and carbamazepine, as well as lamotrigine (as part of multi-organ failure). Valproic acid can cause life-threatening pancreatitis. It can also cause thrombocytopenia. Aplastic anemia and agranulocytosis have been reported with carbamazepine. Gabapentin may cause hyponatremia, which usually develops early in the course of treatment. Topiramate frequently causes concentration difficulties, weight loss, paresthesias, and nephrolithiasis. Carbamazepine, oxcarbazepine, and topiramate may reduce the efficacy of oral contraceptives. Anticonvulsants may increase risk for suicidality (FDA, 2008).

## Alpha-agonists (see also Chapter 5)

Common side effects include dry mouth, drowsiness, dizziness, constipation, and sedation. Children generally experience orthostatic hypotension less than adults do; however, children may be more susceptible to rebound hypertension if these agents are discontinued abruptly.

## Beta-blockers

Common side effects include dizziness, fatigue, bradycardia, mental status changes, gastrointestinal upset, and various skin rashes. Less common – but more serious – adverse events can be bronchospasm and heart failure, both of which may occur more readily in children.

## Anxiolytics (see also Chapter 4)

The benzodiazepines can cause sedation, behavioral disinhibition (similar to that seen with alcohol intoxication), worsening of cognitive functioning, and withdrawal seizures. They also have the potential for being abused or causing dependence. The use of buspirone avoids the abuse and dependence issues, but not side effects.

## Sedative-hypnotics (see also Chapter 11)

Adverse effects from these agents are similar to those seen with the anxiolytics. In addition, their use may not normalize sleep architecture, or can even further disrupt it. Chloral hydrate's main side effects are gastrointestinal, or occasionally cutaneous, including urticaria, purpura, or eczema.

## Antihistamines

The most common side effects are sedation, fatigue, drying of the mucous membranes, dizziness, increased appetite, constipation, and difficulty with urination.

## Opioid antagonists

The most common side effects are nausea and gastrointestinal upset.

## Contraindications

Unless stated otherwise, it is assumed that any medication will have as a contraindication sensitivity to that medication or any of its ingredients.

## Psychostimulants (see also Chapter 5)

Use of these medications is contraindicated in patients who are already experiencing significant levels of anxiety, inner tension, or psychomotor agitation. They should not be used if glaucoma is present. They should also not be used if patients are on MAOIs, or if those medications have been discontinued within the last 2 weeks. Their use in the presence of motor tic disorder or Tourette's disorder is relatively contraindicated (see Chapter 12). Another relative contraindication is a seizure disorder. The use of the mixed amphetamines is also contraindicated if the patient has symptomatic cardiovascular disease, hypertension, or hyperthyroidism.

## Antidepressants (see also Chapter 6)

All of the non-MAOI antidepressants are contraindicated for concurrent use with MAOIs. At least 2 weeks must pass after an MAOI has been discontinued before any other antidepressant can be safely started. Before starting an MAOI, other antidepressants should be stopped at least 2 weeks beforehand (exceptions are venlafaxine, which requires at least 1 week, and fluoxetine, which requires at least 5 weeks). All antidepressants with serotonergic activity (except mirtazapine and venlafaxine) are contraindicated for use with pimozide, the combination of which can greatly prolong the $QT_c$ interval (fluoxetine and paroxetine should not be used concurrently with thioridazine, and nefazodone with carbamazepine, for similar reasons).

Bupropion is contraindicated in patients with a seizure disorder or an eating disorder (which, in combination with bupropion, increases the risk of a seizure).

The MAOI antidepressants should not be used in patients with pheochromocytoma, heart failure or other cardiovascular disease, cerebrovascular disease, or liver disease. There are also several medications which should not be used in combination with the MAOI, especially dextromethorphan, meperidine, and any with sympathomimetic actions.

## Antipsychotics (see also Chapter 8)

The use of clozapine is contraindicated in persons with myeloproliferative disorders, poorly controlled seizure disorders, paralytic ileus, or a prior adverse hematologic reaction to clozapine. The other second-generation antipsychotics have no specific contraindications, except for ziprasidone, which should not be used in persons with congenital long QT syndrome, or concurrently with other medications which have the potential for prolonging the QT interval.

## Mood stabilizers

Lithium should not be used in patients with severe cardiovascular disease, renal disease (unless already on dialysis), dehydration, or sodium depletion (or medications that cause it). Persons with brain damage may be more sensitive to lithium's neurotoxic potential.

Given that carbamazepine has a tricyclic structure, its use with MAOI needs to follow the same guidelines as noted previously for the antidepressants. It should be avoided in persons with prior bone marrow suppression, as well as in individuals with acute intermittent porphyria. Although oxcarbazepine is very closely related to carbamazepine, it does not have specific restrictions to its use (other than known hypersensitivity to the drug itself).

Valproic acid should not be used in the presence of significant hepatic dysfunction or a urea cycle disorder.

There are no specific contraindications for the use of lamotrigine, gabapentin, or topiramate.

## Alpha-agonists (see also Chapter 5)

There are no known specific contraindications to their use.

## Beta-blockers

The major contraindications pertain to the cardiovascular and respiratory systems. The beta-blockers should not be used in patients with sinus bradycardia and greater than first-degree block, asthma, sick sinus syndrome, significant peripheral arterial disease, pheochromocytoma, and right ventricular failure associated with pulmonary hypertension.

## Anxiolytics (see also Chapter 4)

The benzodiazepines should not be used if patients have acute narrow angle glaucoma. Abuse or dependence potential may exclude use in certain individuals. The use of buspirone is contraindicated in combination with an MAOI.

## Sedative-hypnotics (see also Chapter 11)

It is interesting that the hypnotics that are benzodiazepine in nature do not have contraindicated use in persons with glaucoma. Chloral hydrate should not be used in the presence of significant hepatic or renal impairment.

## Antihistamines

Cyproheptadine should not be used with MAOI (due to prolongation of cyproheptadine's inherent anticholinergic effects). Its use should also be avoided in cases of asthma, narrow-angle glaucoma, stenosing peptic ulcer disease, bladder neck obstruction (or other urinary retention), and pyloroduodenal obstruction.

**Table 10.6** Developmental syndromes associated with seizures.

| Syndrome | Rate (approximate %) of seizures |
| --- | --- |
| Angelman | 80 |
| Autism | 20–30[a] |
| Cerebral palsy | 25–50[a] |
| Down | 5–10 |
| Fragile X | 15–20 |
| Neurofibromatosis type 1 | 3–5 |
| Rett | 25–30 |
| Smith–Magenis | 25–50 |
| Sturge–Weber | 72–93 |
| Tuberous sclerosis | 80 |
| Velocardiofacial | 7 |

[a] Correlates with the degree of mental retardation.

## Opioid antagonists

Naltrexone should not be used concurrently with opioid analgesics, or within 7–10 days after discontinuing their use. Its use is also contraindicated in acute hepatitis or liver failure.

## How to use the medications: problem-oriented approaches

Before discussing the use of psychotropic medications in persons with mental retardation, it is important to consider the presence of seizure disorders in various developmental syndromes (Table 10.6). In general, up to one-third of children with mental retardation have some type of epilepsy, and at least one-third of children with epilepsy have some degree of mental retardation.

The coexistence of seizures with intellectual impairment can be problematic in three ways. Firstly, it can cause diagnostic confusion, in that it may be difficult to tell if the patient's emotional, cognitive, and/or behavioral symptoms are from the seizure activity, from the mental retardation itself, and/or from any of the comorbid psychiatric disorders that will be addressed shortly. Secondly, it can present some treatment dilemmas, as some psychotropic medications may affect – or be affected by – anti-epileptic drugs (AEDs). Some psychotropic medications may lower the seizure threshold.

They may also precipitate or exacerbate psychiatric symptoms. Finally, treating comorbid conditions increases the risk of polypharmacy, which increases the chances of undesirable medication effects.

Following are some of the common clinical issues that practitioners face in dealing with their intellectually impaired patients.

## Aggression (see also Chapter 7)

It is important to remember that aggression – i.e. verbal or physical behavior that leads to emotional or physical (person or property) damage – is a *symptom*, not a diagnosis. Its etiology is varied, and often multifactorial. It is one of the most common problems seen in persons with intellectual disabilities, and one of the most frightening. Once medical and substance-related causes are excluded, psychiatric disorders must be identified before specific treatments can be instituted.

The risk for developing aggressive behavior may be higher in certain syndromes associated with lowered IQ, such as Prader–Willi syndrome (PWS), Fetal alcohol syndrome (FAS), Fragile X syndrome (FXS), Smith–Magenis syndrome (SMS), Tuberous sclerosis complex (TSC), Cri-du-chat syndrome (CCS) and, to a lesser extent, Down syndrome (DS).

*Prader–Willi syndrome.* The aggression in PWS is usually described as "temper outbursts," although frank physical acts towards others can be seen. Some of the behaviors may derive from attempts by caregivers to curb the compulsive behaviors (especially related to food) seen in PWS patients. A reasonable first choice would be an SSRI, such as fluoxetine, which may reduce aggressiveness in these patients, even in the absence of depression. Unfortunately, there is the possibility that an SSRI may worsen anger and aggressive behavior; in that case, fluoxetine's long half-life would be especially problematic. An alternative to consider would be an AED with a low potential for weight gain, such as carbamazepine, oxcarbazepine, lamotrigine, or gabapentin. Valproic acid should probably be avoided, due to its tendency to promote weight gain; a similar caution exists for lithium. In patients for whom neither antidepressants nor mood stabilizers have been effective, one may consider using a second-generation antipsychotic. However, as PWS patients are already prone to weight gain, the only available SGAs with low weight-gain potential are clozapine, ziprasidone, and aripiprazole, although risperidone has been reported to have been used successfully with PWS patients. <u>Caveat</u>: No matter which medications are used, low dosing and careful monitoring are in order, as patients with PWS are extremely sensitive to medications, may not metabolize them well, and may have paradoxical reactions.

*Fetal alcohol syndrome.* Patients with FAS display both verbal and physical aggression, which often derives from their poor interpersonal skills, especially during their interactions with authority figures. Comorbidity is quite common in these patients, with elevated rates of ADHD, anxiety, depression, psychotic-like symptoms, and intermittent explosive disorder (IED). Those conditions should be treated first, as their resolution may also diminish or eliminate the aggressive behaviors (see the specific problem sections below for treatment recommendations). For IED symptoms not responsive to other medications, lithium, anticonvulsants, or beta-blockers (especially the lipophilic agents propranolol and metoprolol) may be effective.

*Fragile X syndrome.* The patients with FXS are fairly similar, in terms of symptoms, to those with FAS, and have similar psychiatric comorbidities. The important differences are that in FXS patients there is a risk of seizures in the younger age group, and in about 20% motor tics are present (see "Movement disorders" below). If aggressive behavior persists after treating comorbid conditions, and if a seizure disorder is not present, one should still consider a trial of an AED, followed by lithium. Another option would be a beta-blocker.

*Smith–Magenis syndrome.* The aggression seen in SMS is thought to be related to ADHD symptoms, which are usually severe, and are seen in over 80% of patients. Treating the hyperactivity with stimulants may effectively reduce the aggressivity, but also may not. As these patients also have a high rate of seizure activity (and even higher rates of abnormal EEGs, even in the absence of seizures), a better first choice may be AEDs, especially carbamazepine or valproic acid. Another option would be an SSRI, especially if there is suspicion that the irritability is related to the obsessive-type of anxiety seen in SMS patients (see "Self-injurious behavior" and "Obsessions/compulsions" below). The atypical antipsychotics should probably be avoided, as at least one-half of patients with SMS have hyperlipidemia.

*Tuberous sclerosis complex.* Patients with TSC are indeed complex, given the high rate of seizure disorders, the common occurrence of ADHD symptoms (see "Hyperactivity/impulsivity" below), and cardiac and renal involvement. Aggression in these patients is common, shows wide variation in severity, and does not tend to diminish over time (except for destructive outbursts). As much of the aggressive behavior in TSC is probably related to the seizure disorder, the first step in management should be maximizing the AED regimen. The use of any medication that may affect cardiac conduction should be delayed until the TSC patient has had a thorough cardiac evaluation. About one-half of these patients will have a cardiac rhabdomyoma, and about 20% of those will be associated with arrhythmias.

*Cri-du-chat syndrome.* There is speculation that much of the aggression (towards person and property) seen in CCS derives from the poor or absent language skills that the majority of patients evidence. Hyperactive behavior has been variously reported in these patients, and it seems to diminish with age. If improvement in communication skills does not help to diminish the aggressive behaviors, a cautious trial of stimulants may be indicated (see "Hyperactivity/impulsivity" below).

*Down syndrome.* Children with DS are typically thought of as pleasant and compliant, but, for at least 10%, they can present as oppositional and aggressive. Given that ADHD symptoms are present at rates similar to those seen in control groups, and also given that anxiety, depression, and seizures increase in incidence with increasing age, it is not surprising that the rate of disruptive behaviors in DS children is low. It is unlikely that medications will be needed in any but a few of these patients who do not respond to behavioral interventions. This is fortunate, in that DS patients have higher rates of medical problems (such as hypothyroidism and thrombocytopenia) which would complicate the use of psychotropic agents.

## Self-injurious behavior (SIB)

This can be as disturbing as aggression, because it is aggression – towards the self. It also can derive from any number of etiologies, either single or multiple. The developmental syndromes in which SIB is commonly seen are PWS, FXS, CCS, SMS, Cornelia de Lange syndrome (CdLS), and Lesch–Nyhan syndrome (LNS).

*Prader–Willi syndrome.* Self-injurious behavior is seen in the vast majority of PWS patients. It mostly consists of skin-picking, with some preference for legs, face, and arms; however, other types of self-injury (e.g. head banging) can be seen. As there is a strong obsessive-compulsive component to the self-injury in these patients, treatment should begin with an SSRI. If the patient fails two reasonable trials with an SSRI, low-dose risperidone (starting at 0.5 mg/day) may help. The use of naltrexone – alone or in combination with other medications – has the potential for reducing SIB. One study of adults with PWS demonstrated a significant reduction in skin-picking behaviors with the use of topiramate; its use in younger patients may be considered if other treatments are unsuccessful. Topiramate should be divided into twice-daily dosing, as renal clearance of the drug is increased in pediatric patients.

*Fragile X syndrome.* Onset of SIB in patients with FXS tends to be early in life, and the self-injury has a modest correlation with other problem behaviors. The SIB is usually related to frustration in a task situation. The most common SIB seen is biting of the hands and fingers, followed by hitting of the head and pulling of hair or skin. These behaviors will usually respond to a combination of adequate treatment of comorbid conditions (e.g. ADHD, depression, anxiety) and behavioral interventions.

*Cri-du-chat syndrome.* Self-injury is very common in CCS, with patients engaging in several behaviors, most commonly hitting or banging of the head, biting, or scratching. Stereotypical behaviors (e.g. body rocking, hand waving) are also common, and may share an etiological connection with the SIB. Given that possibility, and also that stereotypies can respond to dopaminergic blockade, treating with low-dose risperidone seems reasonable.

*Smith–Magenis syndrome.* Self-injurious behaviors are seen in essentially all patients with SMS, and tend to increase with age. Hand-biting is far and away the most common form of SIB, followed by self-slapping, head-banging, and picking of the skin and toe – and fingernails (to the point of bleeding). These patients will also stick various objects into body orifices. As there are features of compulsivity, stereotypy, and self-stimulation in SMS patients, trials of an SSRI, an atypical antipsychotic, and/or naltrexone may be necessary.

*Cornelia de Lange syndrome.* Estimates of SIB in CdLS are quite variable. The behaviors themselves are typically of the hitting, banging, biting, or pulling

**Table 10.7** Developmental syndromes commonly associated with ADHD.

| | |
|---|---|
| Angelman syndrome (AS) | Neurofibromatosis type-I (NF-1) |
| Autistic spectrum disorders (ASD) | Smith–Magenis syndrome (SMS) |
| Cri-du-chat syndrome (CCS) | Tuberous sclerosis complex (TSC) |
| Fetal alcohol syndrome (FAS) | Velocardiofacial syndrome(VCFS) |
| Fragile X syndrome (FXS) | Williams syndrome (WS) |

at oneself types. Environmental changes tend to increase the amount of SIB that patients engage in. Patients with CdLS display a curious phenomenon called *self-restraint*, i.e. attempts to limit their self-destructive behaviors (e.g. crowding themselves into a tight space). Self-restraint seems to be correlated with compulsivity; therefore, the first-line treatment for SIB in CdLS patients should be an SSRI.

*Lesch–Nyhan syndrome.* Considered a hallmark of LNS, SIB is eventually seen in almost all individuals with this disorder, although the majority will display it by 3 years of age. Biting of the fingers and hands, lips, and cheeks can be severe, with associated medical complications. Although the use of naltrexone for SIB has yielded some conflicting results, the majority of patients treated with it show a diminution of their self-injurious behaviors. Given the usual severity of self-damage in LNS, a trial of naltrexone seems warranted.

## Hyperactivity/impulsivity (see also Chapter 5)

This is another behavioral complex often seen in the intellectually challenged population. There are numerous syndromes in which ADHD-like signs and symptoms are major contributors to the management difficulties with these patients (Table 10.7 lists several of the more common disorders with ADHD features).

There are some interrelationships between ADHD and epilepsy in the developmentally disabled patient population that have some implications for treatment. Firstly, some of the core symptoms of ADHD may be mimicked by certain types of seizure activity. Secondly, some AEDs may have cognitive and/or behavioral side effects, which may also mimic ADHD. Thirdly, concurrent pharmacotherapy for both conditions can lead to adverse medicine–medicine interactions. Fourthly, patients with ADHD may be at higher risk of developing unprovoked seizures. Finally, some medications that are used to treat ADHD have the potential for lowering the seizure threshold.

Regarding the epileptogenic potential of psychotropic medications, contrary to previous beliefs, methylphenidate (MPH) appears to be safe to use in developmentally disabled patients with comorbid ADHD and a seizure disorder. The seizure disorder should be well-controlled and contraindicated conditions (e.g. psychosis) should be excluded before MPH is started. Other stimulant medications (i.e. the amphetamines) may also be safe to use in this population, but there is little research data to inform decision-making.

Alternatives to the psychostimulants for ADHD include certain antidepressants, alpha-agonists, atomoxetine, and modafinil. The antidepressant used for ADHD with the highest risk of inducing seizures is bupropion, and venlafaxine and the tricyclic antidepressants (TCAs) have moderate risk (seizure risk increases with total daily dose for all of these agents). Clonidine may cause seizures in an overdose situation; it is unknown whether it, or guanfacine, increases seizure risk at normal therapeutic doses. There is no information on atomoxetine and seizure risk; however, given that it increases CNS levels of norepinephrine, it has theoretical epileptogenic potential at high doses. There are some data that suggest that modafinil's ability to enhance cognitive functioning may extend to counteracting the cognitive dulling effects of the AEDs. It may also have anticonvulsant activity. Modafinil may therefore be a better and safer agent to use in the intellectually disabled patient with comorbid seizure disorder and ADHD.

## Sleep disturbances (see also Chapter 11)

These are ubiquitous problems in those with cognitive disabilities. They are especially prominent in patients with PWS, AS, DS, FXS, SMS, CdLS, and WS. It is important to treat sleep problems, as they may contribute to cognitive and behavioral problems.

The increased incidence of excessive daytime sleepiness in PWS patients is likely secondary to sleep apnea or hypothalamic dysfunction, and sleep-onset REM is suggestive of narcolepsy. The former condition may be treated with continuous positive airway pressure (CPAP), and both may be treated with modafinil.

The sleep disorders in AS are both dyssomnias (e.g. insomnia) and parasomnias, especially those involving Stage IV sleep, such as sleep terrors, sleepwalking, and enuresis. Melatonin, starting at 0.5 mg before bed, can be quite effective in improving sleep quality.

Patients with DS frequently have obstructive sleep apnea. They also have difficulty in maintaining sleep, not all of which can be attributed to the apnea. If the use of CPAP is clinically indicated, but does not solve the sleep problem, medication options include low doses of melatonin, ramelteon (a prescription melatonin receptor agonist), or trazodone.

The patients with FXS also have difficulty with initiating and maintaining sleep. The interventions suggested for DS patients would also be appropriate for FXS patients. In addition, the use of clonidine for sleep is an option, especially considering the high rate of ADHD in that population.

The sleep disturbances in SMS include delayed sleep onset, frequent nocturnal awakenings, difficulty re-establishing sleep, enuresis, and daytime sleepiness and napping. Melatonin appears to be the medication of choice, pending further research.

There are no pharmacologic agents that are specifically recommended for the sleep problems in CdLS. However, given that the sleep symptoms are similar to those seen in other developmental syndromes, it seems reasonable to try melatonin first in those patients.

The sleep disorder in WS is unusual, in that there are excessive periodic limb movements during sleep, which contribute to the other symptoms of abnormal sleep. Unlike most of the other sleep disorders linked to developmental syndromes, the use of benzodiazepines, such as clonazepam, is actually indicated for the periodic limb movements, which respond fairly dramatically to this treatment.

## Eating disturbances

Issues with food intake and/or body weight are problematic in persons with AS, PWS, DS, ASD, and WS. The most common types of problems in this area are overeating, extreme selectivity, and food refusal associated with poor appetite. The initial approach should be with a behavioral plan. In the case of poor appetite, once medical and psychiatric issues have been treated, and eating has not improved, a trial of an appetite stimulant, such as the antihistamine cyproheptadine, may be initiated.

*Angelman syndrome.* Feeding problems in the younger AS patient are often replaced by an excessive pickiness about food, increased appetite, and even the eating of nonfood items. Attempts to modify the eating habits may provoke anger and aggressive behavior (see "Aggression" above).

*Prader–Willi syndrome.* The hallmark of PWS is a seemingly insatiable hunger, with associated preoccupation with food, hyperphagia, and a tendency to gain excessive weight. As previously noted in AS, patients with PWS may likewise become upset whenever efforts are undertaken to change their eating habits to reduce caloric intake. A trial of fluoxetine may be indicated, especially if nonfood obsessions are present (see "Obsessions/compulsions" below). If self-injury in the form of skin picking is severe enough to warrant a trial of medication (see "Self-injurious behavior" above), topiramate may be a good choice, as it may have additional benefit as an appetite suppressant. Psychostimulants should not be used as anorectic agents, as their effects are inconsistent and they also increase the risk of pulmonary hypertension.

*Down syndrome.* The weight gain seen in persons with DS is a result of a lowered resting metabolic rate that is not secondary to hypothyroidism. The intervention of choice is a well-planned regimen of diet and exercises that should begin early in life. Pharmacologic agents can be useful adjuncts when used to treat other conditions (such as anxiety or depression) that may interfere with compliance with lifestyle modifications.

*Autistic spectrum disorders (ASD).* Children with an ASD (see also Chapter 9) tend to be rigid in their thinking and ritualistic in their behaviors. This is also true in the area of eating, where there are often concerns over food refusal and food selectivity. Medications may be necessary in cases in which food intake is low enough to compromise nutrition and health, and if one or more psychiatric disorders are determined to be the cause(s).

*Williams syndrome.* The early feeding problems in WS, and subsequent poor weight gain and linear growth are the result of the inherent metabolic and endocrine abnormalities in this syndrome. Weight gain can be further compromised by decreased appetite and eating secondary to a psychiatric disorder (e.g. anxiety), or to side effects from medications used to treat other disorders (e.g. ADHD). Efforts should be made to identify all treatable psychiatric conditions, and medications should be chosen carefully to avoid adverse effects on growth.

# Obsessions/compulsions

Obsessions/compulsions (see also Chapter 4) are common clinical features in PWS, FXS, DS, ASD, VCFS, and WS. The diagnosis of obsessive-compulsive disorder (OCD) can be made with either obsessions or compulsions alone, although they frequently co-occur.

*Prader–Willi syndrome.* Patients with PWS may have difficulty recognizing and describing obsessional thinking, which is a challenge for the clinician evaluating for OCD. However, compulsive activity is common and often quite striking in these patients. Hoarding behavior can include nonfood items; excessive time can also be spent on arranging objects, routines, and/or asking questions and sharing information. If the ritualistic activities interfere with more important functions, or if attempts to interrupt the behaviors cause distress, the child should be treated for OCD. The treatment can be any one of the SSRIs that are approved for OCD.

*Fragile X syndrome.* Characteristic OCD-like symptoms in FXS patients include repeating words and phrases, strict adherence to routines, arranging items, and repetitious movements of body parts. The rates of these behaviors increases with the degree of autistic thinking present. The rationale and approach to treatment is similar to that in PWS, i.e. the use of serotonergic antidepressants.

*Down syndrome.* The OCD-like symptoms in DS patients tend to be more subtle than those seen in the other developmental syndromes described in this chapter. What is commonly described as "stubbornness" can actually be indecisiveness and slowness related to obsessional thinking. There is a greater than average risk of comorbid ASD with DS, and presence of the former may confer a greater risk for OCD-type symptoms in DS. As noted previously, the SSRIs should be tried first as treatment for the obsessive-compulsive features.

*Autistic spectrum disorders.* The symptoms of OCD and their treatments are consistent with those seen in other disorders, such as FXS.

*Velocardiofacial syndrome.* The diagnosis of OCD can be made in about one-third of patients with VCFS. There is early onset of symptoms, and the types of obsessions and compulsions are similar to those seen in the normal IQ population with OCD, such as concerns about contamination and bodily functioning and excessive cleaning. There can also be hoarding and excessive questioning as seen in other developmental disorders. Response to fluoxetine is generally good.

*Williams syndrome.* The patients with WS display preoccupations with ideas or activities, and utter words and phrases repetitively. These problem areas reach a high level of intensity early in life, with the verbal perseveration tending to diminish with age. As discussed with the other syndromes, pharmacologic treatment is considered if symptom intensity is disruptive or distressing, and is not responding to behavioral interventions. The SSRIs remain the medications of choice.

## Other anxiety disorders

Anxiety (see also Chapter 4) can be a significant component of the clinical picture in DS, FXS, FAS, PWS, neurofibromatosis type-1 (NF-1), velocardiofacial syndrome (VCFS), and WS.

*Down syndrome.* The prevalence of anxiety disorders in DS children is not significantly higher than that seen in matched control groups. Anxiety does increase, however, with increasing age in this population. Given that pediatricians are sometimes the default physicians for these patients, it is important to screen for anxiety disorders in older adolescents and adults with DS. If identified, anxiety can be treated with buspirone or an SSRI, the latter also able to treat comorbid depression that may be present (see "Depression" below).

*Fragile X syndrome.* Anxiety disorders are not uncommon in FXS patients, especially panic disorder and social phobia. The main medication options are either an SSRI or buspirone; benzodiazepines should be avoided, if possible, as they can cause behavioral disinhibition in persons with FXS.

*Fetal alcohol syndrome.* Children with FAS who also have mental retardation (from mild up to moderate–severe) have higher rates of anxiety than age-matched controls. By adulthood, about one-third of FAS patients will suffer with panic attacks. The SSRIs are the medications of choice. Use of benzodiazepines is relatively contraindicated, given their cross-tolerance with alcohol and the increased risk of dependency in FAS patients.

*Prader–Willi syndrome.* About 70% of patients with PWS, at all ages, experience anxiety *not* related to food. Low-dose SSRI (e.g. fluoxetine) or buspirone can be used; careful monitoring is required.

*Neurofibromatosis type-1.* The most common type of anxiety problem in persons with NF-1 is social anxiety. If not responsive to cognitive and behavioral interventions, the social anxiety can be treated with either sertraline or paroxetine (see Chapter 1 for more on psychological treatments).

*Velocardiofacial syndrome.* Patients with VCFS experience phobic anxiety, which becomes more severe at the time of puberty. Cognitive–behavioral therapy (CBT) is the treatment of choice for simple phobias. However, if the patient's anxiety is so severe that he/she cannot engage in the therapy, then a cautious trial of low-dose, short-term benzodiazepine might be indicated.

*Williams syndrome.* Generalized anxiety, with a strong anticipatory component, is seen in over one-half of persons with WS. Some degree of phobic anxiety is seen in nearly all of these patients, accompanied by excessive worrying. Escitalopram – with or without CBT – would be a good first-choice.

## Depression
Depression (see also Chapter 6) can be seen in any developmental disorder, but is more common in DS, FAS, FXS, NF-1, PWS, and VCFS.

*Down syndrome.* Similar to the rates of anxiety, depression in DS patients also increases with age. The SSRIs are the medications of choice, given the likely presence of comorbid OCD and/or other anxiety disorders. If not responsive to the SSRIs, the depression can be treated with any other type of antidepressant, with the exception of bupropion (seizure risk).

*Fetal alcohol syndrome.* About one-half of children with FAS will become clinically depressed, and almost one-quarter will make a suicide attempt. Any antidepressant can be used to treat depression in this population.

*Fragile X syndrome.* The rate of depression is somewhat related to genetic status, as it is more likely to be experienced by female carriers (i.e. with greater than 100 CGG-trinucleotide repeats) and males with the full mutation. Medication recommendations are similar to those given for the treatment of depression in DS.

*Neurofibromatosis type-1.* Based on parental reports, patients with NF-1 seem to be at higher risk for depression. If criteria are met for treatment, any antidepressant can be used, although bupropion should be at the bottom of the list, given the risk (albeit low) of seizures in NF-1 patients.

*Prader–Willi syndrome.* The depression in PWS is often experienced as sadness and a feeling that life is not worth living. There is an inverse relationship between body-mass index (BMI) and level of depression, such that worsening of depression can be anticipated as dietary restrictions lead to loss of body weight. Other factors that increase the rate of depression are increasing age and male sex (in the deletion sub-type). Any antidepressant can be used to treat depression in this population. Serotonergic medications may increase appetite, so serial body weights should be measured.

*Velocardiofacial syndrome.* Patients with VCFS have elevated rates of mood disorders, especially major depression and bipolar disorder. The risk of depression increases with age. Bupropion may have less risk (compared with other antidepressants) of provoking a "manic switch" in bipolar disorder. The risk of developing a seizure disorder is low in VCFS patients, so a cautious trial of bupropion is warranted if the patient has a history of symptoms suggestive of bipolar disorder, or has a family history of that illness. In the case of documented manic or hypomanic symptoms in the patient's past, the treatment of depression should follow the recommendations established for bipolar depression (see Chapter 6).

## Psychosis
Although uncommon, psychotic-like symptoms (see also Chapter 8) may be seen in FAS, FXS, VCFS, and PWS.

*Fetal alcohol syndrome.* The risk of a person with FAS developing a psychotic disorder may increase with age (40% of adults in one study). Paranoid thinking may be present, even in the absence of overt psychosis. Treatment with risperidone is usually effective, and the potential side effects of increased appetite and weight are of minimal concern in most FAS patients (who tend to be of slight body build).

*Fragile X syndrome.* Although psychosis may be seen in patients with FXS, it is a rare occurrence. It may be treated with any of the atypical antipsychotics, except clozapine, which lowers the seizure threshold.

*Velocardiofacial syndrome.* Psychosis is present in about one-third of patients with VCFS. There is some question as to whether it may be comorbid with bipolar disorder in this population. A small percentage of patients with childhood-onset schizophrenia will also have VCFS. The atypical antipsychotics (except for clozapine) are also used for bipolar disorder, so they can treat psychotic symptoms as well as the mood disorder, if present.

*Prader Willi syndrome.* Patients with PWS can develop a host of psychotic symptoms, including delusions. The risk of a PWS patient becoming psychotic actually decreases with an increase in BMI. Therefore, patients who are participating in a medically supervised weight loss regimen should be monitored closely for emergent psychotic symptoms. If medication is needed to treat the psychotic symptoms, the choices are either ziprasidone or aripiprazole, as they have the lowest incidence of weight gain, a major concern in patients with PWS.

## Movement disorders

The main concerns regarding psychotropic medication use in movement disorders (see also Chapter 12) are that it may exacerbate the abnormal movements seen in various developmental syndromes or may interact with medications used to control the movements, thus increasing the risk for adverse side effects.

Abnormal movements may be a major focus of clinical intervention, or may interfere with other therapeutic measures, such as social skills training.

Abnormal movements and/or body posturing may be seen in AS, FXS, cerebral palsy (CP), SLOS, SMS, and LNS.

*Angelman syndrome.* The abnormal movements displayed by patients with AS are noted to be jerky, with hand-flapping and myoclonic tremors of the fingers. Gait is ataxic.

*Fragile X syndrome.* The significant abnormal movements seen in FXS patients are tics, which occur in about 20% of individuals.

*Cerebral palsy.* The typical motor abnormalities of CP are well-known to pediatricians. About 60% of these patients will have some degree of intellectual impairment.

*Smith–Lemli–Opitz syndrome.* In slightly more than one-half of patients with SLOS will be seen an exaggerated arching of the head and trunk. This occurs before the age of 5 years, and diminishes with age.

*Smith–Magenis syndrome.* Patients with SMS display a peculiar motor behavior called *self-hugging*, wherein they literally hug their own torso. This tends to be quite repetitive, and can occur hundreds of times in a day.

*Lesch–Nyhan syndrome.* Extra-pyramidal symptoms can be seen in LNS during the first year of life.

## How to monitor the medication (including what tests are needed)

### Psychostimulants (see also Chapter 5)

In cases of prolonged treatment, periodic complete blood count (CBC), with differential and platelet count, are recommended. Blood pressure and pulse should be checked at each medication visit, as both values can increase with stimulant treatment. Height and weight should be measured per routine schedule, and any significant slowing, stoppage, or loss should prompt discontinuation and medical evaluation.

### Antidepressants (see also Chapter 6)

No routine laboratory tests (including serum sodium) are required for any of these medications. However, venlafaxine may raise serum cholesterol, such that checking levels should be considered during prolonged treatment. The selegiline patch infrequently elevates liver function test values; routine testing is not recommended.

## Antipsychotics (see also Chapter 8)

It is important that the patient's height, weight, BMI, blood pressure, pulse, and fasting glucose and lipids be measured before starting treatment with these agents. A baseline examination for abnormal neuromotor (extrapyramidal) signs is suggested. The only atypical antipsychotic that requires baseline and follow-up ECGs is ziprasidone. All of these parameters, as well as a serum prolactin level (especially in females), should be rechecked during the course of treatment.

## Mood stabilizers

Before starting lithium obtain baseline electrolytes, BUN, creatinine, thyroid function tests, WBC, and urine specific gravity; repeat 1 or 2 times/year, once the patient is stabilized. A serum lithium trough level (10–12 hours after last dose) should be measured 4–5 days after starting the medication, 4–5 days after any dosage increase, and every 3–6 months during the maintenance phase.

In patients on valproic acid, baseline and follow-up (every 6–12 months) AST, ALT, LDH, and CBC should be measured. The drug level should be checked 1–2 weeks after initiation or after each dosage increase, and also every 3–6 months during maintenance.

The monitoring for carbamazepine is essentially the same as for valproic acid.

No specific laboratory monitoring is required when using lamotrigine, gabapentin, or topiramate.

## Alpha-agonists (see also Chapter 5)

Blood pressure should be monitored for hypotension and rebound hypertension. No laboratory studies are required.

## Beta-blockers

Blood pressure and pulse should be routinely monitored. There is rarely a need for laboratory testing for this class. Propranolol can sometimes cause elevations in serum potassium, AST, ALT, and alkaline phosphatase in hypertensive patients. Pindolol can also occasionally elevate AST, ALT, and alkaline phosphatase, as well as LDH and uric acid.

**Table 10.8** Summary of medication recommendations.

| Problem | 1st choice | 2nd choice | 3rd choice |
|---|---|---|---|
| **Aggression in:** | | | |
| CCS | Stimulant | RISP | Mood stabilizer |
| DS | SSRI | 2nd SSRI | Mood stabilizer |
| FAS (with IED) | Lithium | AED | Beta-blocker |
| FXS (with IED) | AED | Lithium | Beta-blocker |
| PWS | SSRI or AED | AED or SSRI | SGA |
| SMS | AED | SSRI (or stimulant) | Stimulant (or SSRI) |
| TSC | AED | 2nd AED | Stimulant |
| **Self–injury in:** | | | |
| CCS | RISP | 2nd SGA | 3rd SGA? |
| CdLS | SSRI | 2nd SSRI | 3rd SSRI ? |
| FXS | SSRI (or stimulant) | Stimulant (or SSRI) | SGA ? |
| LNS | Naltrexone | SSRI ? | SGA ? |
| PWS | SSRI | 2nd SSRI | RISP; Topiramate ? |
| SMS | SSRI (or SGA) | SGA (or SSRI) | Naltrexone ? |
| **ADHD in:** | Seizure +/−: | | |
| See Table 10.7 | Modafinil/stimulant | Stimulant | Alpha-agonist ? |
| **Poor sleep in:** | | | |
| AS | Melatonin | Ramelteon ? | |
| CdLS | Melatonin | Ramelteon ? | |
| DS | Melatonin | Ramelteon | Trazodone |
| FXS | Melatonin | Ramelteon | Clonidine |
| PWS | Modafinil | Stimulant ? | |
| SMS | Melatonin | Ramelteon ? | |
| WS | Clonazepam | 2nd Benzodiazepine | |
| **Eating/feeding in:** | | | |
| AS | There are no specific medications for the eating problems in | | |
| ASD | these conditions. Psychiatric disorders should be identified | | |
| DS | and treated – in coordination with other interventions – to try | | |
| WS | and normalize eating behaviors. Cyproheptadine may act as | | |
| | an appetite stimulant. | | |
| PWS | Fluoxetine | Topiramate? | |
| **OCD in:** | | | |
| ASD | OCD symptoms in all of these conditions should be treated | | |
| DS | with one of the SSRIs approved for use in OCD. They are | | |
| FXS | fluoxetine, sertraline, paroxetine, and fluvoxamine. Keep | | |
| PWS | trying them until one works. Fluvoxamine tends to have | | |
| VCFS | more side effects than the others. For treatment-resistant | | |
| WS | cases, refer to Chapter 3 for guidance. | | |

**Table 10.8** *(cont.)*

| Problem | 1st choice | 2nd choice | 3rd choice |
|---|---|---|---|
| **Anxiety in:** | | | |
| DS | SSRI (or Buspirone) | Buspirone (or SSRI) | Another SSRI |
| FAS | SSRI | 2nd SSRI | 3rd SSRI |
| FXS | SSRI (or Buspirone) | Buspirone (or SSRI) | Another SSRI |
| NF-1 | Sertraline | Paroxetine | Another SSRI ? |
| PWS | SSRI (or Buspirone) | Buspirone (or SSRI) | Another SSRI |
| VCFS | Benzodiazepine ? | | |
| WS | Escitalopram | 2nd SSRI | 3rd SSRI |
| **Depression in:** | | | |
| DS | SSRI | 2nd SSRI | NonSSRI[a] |
| FAS | Any antidepressant | 2nd antidepressant | 3rd antidepressant |
| FXS | SSRI | 2nd SSRI | NonSSRI[a] |
| NF-1 | Any antidepressant[b] | 2nd antidepressant[b] | 3rd antidepressant[b] |
| PWS | Any antidepressant | 2nd antidepressant | 3rd antidepressant |
| VCFS | Buproplon ? | 2nd antidepressant | 3rd antidepressant |
| **Psychosis in:** | | | |
| FAS | RISP | 2nd SGA | 3rd SGA |
| FXS | SGA | 2nd SGA | 3rd SGA |
| PWS | Ziprasidone | Aripiprazole | RISP |
| VCFS | SGA | 2nd SGA | 3rd SGA |

AS, Angelman syndrome; ASD, Autistic spectrum disorder; CCS, Cri-du-chat syndrome; CdLS, Cornelia de Lange syndrome; DS, Down syndrome; FAS, Fetal alcohol syndrome; FXS, Fragile X syndrome; IED, Intermittent explosive disorder; LNS, Lesch–Nyhan syndrome; NF-1, Neurofibromatosis type-1; PWS, Prader–Willi syndrome; SMS, Smith-Magenis syndrome; TSC, Tuberous sclerosis complex; VCFS, Velocardiofacial syndrome; WS, Williams syndrome; AED, anti-epileptic drug; SSRI, selective serotonin reuptake inhibitor; RISP, Risperidone; SGA, Second-generation antipsychotic.

[a] With the exception of bupropion; [b] bupropion should be considered last.

## Anxiolytics (see also Chapter 4)

For patients on long-term therapy with a benzodiazepine, periodic blood testing of the WBC (to check for neutropenia) and liver function tests (to check for elevated bilirubin or LDH) are advised.

## Sedative-hypnotics (see also Chapter 11)

No routine laboratory tests are recommended for this class of medications.

## Antihistamines
No routine laboratory tests are recommended for this class of medications.

## Opioid antagonists
Baseline liver function tests and a urine drug screen for opiates should be obtained before initiating treatment with naltrexone. There is a greater risk of hepatocellular damage with increasing doses of naltrexone, therefore liver functions should be re-assessed after each increase in dosage, or any time there is clinical suspicion of hepatic involvement.

## Summary

Table 10.8 provides a summary of the medication recommendations in this chapter.

SELECTED BIBLIOGRAPHY

Antochi R, Stavrakaki C, Emery PC. 2003. Psychopharmacological treatments in persons with dual diagnosis of psychiatric disorders and developmental disabilities. *Postgrad. Med. J.*, 79:139–46.

Calles JL. 2008. Use of psychotropic medications in children with developmental disabilities. *Pediatr. Clin. N. Am.*, 55: in press.

Einfeld SL, Tonge BJ, Rees VW. 2001. Longitudinal course of behavioral and emotional problems in Williams syndrome. *Am. J. Ment. Retard.*, 106(1):73–81.

Hagerman RJ. 1999. Psychopharmacological interventions in Fragile X syndrome, Fetal Alcohol syndrome, Prader-Willi syndrome, Angelman syndrome, Smith-Magenis syndrome, and Velocardiofacial syndrome. *Ment. Retard. Dev. Disabil. Res. Rev.*, 5:305–13.

Handen BL, Gilchrist R. 2006. Practitioner review: psychopharmacology in children and adolescents with mental retardation. *J. Child. Psychol. Psychiatry*, 47(9):871–82.

Kayl AE, Moore BD. 2000. Behavioral phenotype of Neurofibromatosis, Type 1. *Ment. Retard. Dev. Disabil. Res. Rev.*, 6:117–24.

Matson JL, Bamburg JW, Mayville EA, Pinkston J, Bielecki J, Kuhn D. 2000. Psychopharmacology and mental retardation: a 10 year review (1990–1999). *Res. Dev. Disabil.*, 21:263–96.

Persad V, Thompson MD, Percy ME. 2003. Epilepsy and developmental disability Part I: Developmental disorders in which epilepsy may be comorbid. *J. Dev. Disabil.*, 10(2):123–51.

Pisani F, Oteri G, Costa C, Di Raimondo G, Di Perri R. 2002. Effects of psychotropic drugs on seizure threshold. *Drug. Safety*, 25(2):91–110.

Steinhausen H-C, Von Gontard A, Spohr HL *et al.* 2002. Behavioral phenotypes in four mental retardation syndromes: fetal alcohol syndrome, Prader-Willi syndrome, fragile X syndrome, and tuberous sclerosis. *Am. J. Med. Genet.*, 111(4):381–7.

Thompson MD, Persad V, Hwang P, Percy ME. 2003. Epilepsy and developmental disability Part II: Epilepsies in which developmental and psychiatric disorders may be comorbid. *J. Dev. Disabil.*, 10(2):153–74.

www.fda.gov/medwatch/safety/2008/safety08.htm#Antiepileptic

# Sleep disorders in children and adolescents

## 11

## ■ Introduction

Human life can be divided into three specific stages of consciousness: *wake, non-REM (rapid eye movement) sleep,* and *REM sleep* (Table 11.1). The quality of life during the wakeful stage is heavily dependent on the quality of REM and non-REM sleep experienced, whether during childhood, adolescence, or adulthood. The most restorative sleep is delta sleep (slow wave sleep or deep sleep) that occurs in Stages 3 and 4 of non-REM sleep; it is during these stages that one is the most difficult to waken. Individuals waken during REM sleep, but the state of being awake is normally so brief that it is not recalled later when in the true wake state. Rapid eye movement and generalized muscle atonia are characteristic of REM sleep; diaphragmatic movements and erections are the only muscle movements not inhibited.

Sleep architecture changes from infancy to the adulthood years, and as children mature their sleep patterns begin to look more like adult patterns (Table 11.2). Such changes involve shorter duration of sleep, longer cycles of sleep, reduced requirement for sleep in the daytime, and less REM sleep (that constitutes half of sleep in newborns). Daytime napping is common in children 1.5–5 years of age and becomes less important in older children and adolescents unless there is interruption of normal nocturnal sleep stages. There is reduced total nocturnal sleep from infancy to late adolescence, and as adolescence emerges, there is a shift to later bedtime or sleep onset hour. Also, there is a 40% reduction in the REM sleep stage from ages 10 to 20 years. Non-REM:REM sleep ratios are approximately 75%:25% in healthy young

**Table 11.1** Stages of human consciousness.

1. Being awake
2. Non-REM sleep (rapid eye movement)
   a. Stage 1 Sleep (transition of wake and sleep): light sleep
   b. Stage 2 Sleep (starts true sleep state)
   c. Stage 3: first part of deep sleep (also called delta or slow wave sleep)
   d. Stage 4: second part of deep sleep
3. REM Sleep (rapid eye movement with generalized muscle atonia)

**Table 11.2** Normal sleep duration in pediatric stages.[a]

1. Newborn: 16–20 hours per 24 hours
2. Infants: 14–15 hours per 24 hours
3. Toddlers (1–3 years): 12 hours per 24 hours
4. Pre-School Children (3–5 years): 11–12 hours/24 hours
5. School age Children (6–12 years): 10–11 hours/24 hours
6. Adolescents: 9 hours per 24 hours

[a] Individual variations in exact amounts occur.
*Source:* Owens, JA. 2006. Sleep disorders in children and adolescents. In
Greydanus DE, Patel DR, Pratt HD (Eds.) *Behavioral Pediatrics, 2nd edn.*
New York: iUniverse Publishers, pp. 236–64.

adults, and healthy adolescents need approximately 9 hours of nocturnal
sleep for optimal functioning, though individual variation is noted. There
is a normal pattern of several non-REM and REM sleep cycles during the
night with brief arousal periods that change from 7–10 times in infancy
to 4–6 cycles in adolescence and adulthood. The sleep and wake cycles are
regulated by many factors, including the internal biologic clock mechanism
(endogenous circadian rhythm). The internal circadian clock is affected by
exposure to light (i.e. turns off the endogenous production of melatonin)
and dark (i.e. turns on endogenous melatonin production). This internal
clock is somewhat responsive to external stimuli or "zeitgebers," such as an
alarm clock or timing of meals.

Though still early in its existence, the study of sleep problems has identified a number of sleep disorders, both primary and secondary (Table 11.3).

Abnormal sleep patterns and disorders are noted in 25–50% of children
and adolescents, with widespread effects on their medical and mental
health functioning. Any child or adolescent can develop abnormal sleep
patterns, including those with a *chronic medical condition, developmental
disorder*, and *psychiatric disorder* (Table 11.4).

**Table 11.3** Sleep disorders.

1. Insomnia
    a. Sleep onset association disorder (delayed sleep phase disorder)
    b. Limit setting sleep disorder
    c. Adjustment sleep disorder
    d. Psychophysiologic insomnia
2. Excessive daytime sleepiness
3. Narcolepsy
4. Klein–Levin syndrome
5. Post-traumatic hypersomnolence
6. Parasomnias
    a. Rhythmic movement disorders (i.e. head banging, head rolling, body rocking)
    b. Bruxism
    c. Sleep talking
    d. Nightmares
    e. Sleep terrors (pavor nocturnus)
    f. Sleep walking (somnambulism)
    g. Nocturnal enuresis
7. Sleep-disordered breathing
    a. Obstructive sleep apnea/ hypopnea syndrome (OSAHS)
8. Restless legs syndrome (periodic limb movement disorder)

*Sources:* Owens, JA. 2006. Sleep disorders in children and adolescents. In Greydanus DE, Patel DR, Pratt HD (Eds.) *Behavioral Pediatrics, 2nd edn.* New York: iUniverse Publishers, pp. 236–64.
Schuen JN. 2006. Sleep disorders in the adolescent. In Greydanus DE, Patel DR, Pratt HD (Eds.) *Essential Adolescent Medicine.* New York: McGraw-Hill Medical Publishers, pp. 281–97.

Chronic medical disorders may interfere with normal sleep patterns because of such issues as pain, frequent hospitalizations (with regular nocturnal interruptions), depression, anxiety, family dynamics, medications that disrupt sleep, and others. A major contributor to abnormal sleep patterns in many children and adolescents is the use of many medications (prescription and over-the-counter) that can have adverse effects on sleep functioning (Table 11.5). Medications can interfere with normal sleep patterns in many ways, such as inducing increased nocturnal arousals or daytime sedation as well as worsening obstructive sleep apnea or restless legs syndrome.

Many psychiatric disorders interfere with sleep, as listed in Table 11.4. For example, at least half of children and adolescents with attention deficit/hyperactivity disorder (ADHD) have sleep problems that include

**Table 11.4** Disorders with increased incidence of sleep disorders.

1. Chronic medical disorders
   a. Asthma
   b. Cystic fibrosis
   c. Hyperthyroidism
   d. Organ failure (i.e. liver, kidney)
   e. Gastroesophageal reflux
2. Psychiatric disorders
   a. Attention deficit/hyperactivity disorder (ADHD)
   b. Mood disorders
   c. Anxiety disorders
   d. Conduct disorder
   e. Oppositional defiant disorder
   f. Schizophrenia
   g. Others
3. Developmental disorders
   a. Autistic spectrum disorders
   b. Severe mental retardation
   c. Angelman's syndrome
   d. Rett's syndrome
   e. Smith–Magenis syndrome
   f. Down syndrome
   g. Prader–Willi syndrome
   h. Others
4. Fatal familial insomnia (noted in adults)
5. Neuromuscular disorders
   a. Myotonic dystrophy
   b. Duchenne's muscular dystrophy
6. Medications (prescription and over-the-counter) (see Table 11.5)

insomnia, incomplete sleep, and frequent nocturnal awakenings. This pattern of sleep dysfunction may be due to effects of stimulant medications often used to treat ADHD and/or disorders (as depression, anxiety, or oppositional defiant disorder) that are associated with ADHD. Children and adolescents with ADHD may be placed on additional medications to help with insomnia, such as sedating antidepressants, antihistamines, and alpha agonists (Table 11.6).

The evaluation of sleep problems or disorders in children and adolescents begins with a careful history looking for potential sleep abnormalities. Pertinent questions include asking about the regular time of sleep onset, duration of nocturnal sleep, frequency of sleep awakenings, and the

**Table 11.5** Medications interfering with normal sleep patterns.

| Drug | Sleep effect |
| --- | --- |
| Alcohol | Insomnia due to delayed sleep onset |
| Anticonvulsants | Sedation during the day |
| Antihistamines (first-generation) diphenhydramine hydroxyzine chlorpheniramine | Daytime sleepiness; lowers efficiency |
| Antidepressants | |
| SSRI | Activating effects with sleep interruption |
| TCA | Sleepiness in the day due to slow wave sleep blunting |
| Caffeine | Insomnia due to delayed sleep onset |
| Corticosteroids | Stimulating effects leading to insomnia |
| Opioids | Daytime sleepiness, insomnia, nightmares, worsening of obstructive sleep apnea |
| Nicotine (tobacco) | Insomnia due to delayed sleep onset |
| Stimulants methylphenidate dextroamphetamine | Stimulant effects with insomnia (delayed sleep onset) |
| Theophylline | Delayed sleep onset, increased arousals during sleep |

SSRI, selective serotonin reuptake inhibitor; TCA, tricyclic antidepressant.
*Source:* Owens, JA. 2006. Sleep disorders in children and adolescents. In Greydanus DE, Patel DR, Pratt HD (Eds.) *Behavioral Pediatrics, 2nd edn.* New York: iUniverse Publishers, pp. 236–64.

**Table 11.6** Sedating medications used to treat sleep dysfunction in ADHD. Medications are taken at bedtime.

1. Alpha-2 agonists: Clonidine 0.1–0.3 mg
2. Tricyclic antidepressant (TCA): Imipramine, others, 50–75 mg
3. Other antidepressants: Trazodone 25–50 mg
4. Exogenous Melatonin 3–6 mg
5. Selective serotonin reuptake inhibitor (SSRI): Paroxetine 20–30 mg
6. Mirtazapine 7.5–15 mg

presence of such problems as daytime sleepiness and excessive snoring (or other evidence of sleep-disordered breathing). A careful physical examination may reveal evidence of excessive daytime sleepiness (i.e. very tired patient in the office during daytime hours), enlarged tonsils, and others.

Much information can be obtained from a *sleep diary* kept by the patient (with the help of parents in the younger patient) that can be used to identify abnormal patterns of the sleep-awake cycle.

Referral to a local sleep center can be very helpful to have sleep experts continue with a careful history and examinations and provide such useful tools as *actigraphy* and a *sleep lab study*. Actigraphy involves wearing a wrist-watch size device (actigraph) on the wrist or ankle for days to weeks. A sleep lab evaluation takes a video recording of the patient while sleeping and involves a wide range of measurements, including electrocardiogram (2 lead ECG), heart rate, electroencephalogram (EEG), chin and tibial movements (EMG), oronasal flow, chest as well as abdominal movements, oxy-hemoglobin saturations, end-tidal carbon dioxide levels, and others.

A number of sleep disorders will now be discussed.

# ■ Insomnia

The term *insomnia* is a symptom referring to the inability to fall asleep and is not a specific diagnosis. It can be due to a wide range of factors, including chronic poor sleep hygiene, effect of medications or illicit drugs, obstructive sleep apnea, and others. As noted in Table 11.3, a number of insomnia disorders can be classified as *sleep onset association disorder (delayed sleep phase disorder), limit setting sleep disorder, adjustment sleep disorder, psychophysiologic insomnia,* and *altitude insomnia.*

*Sleep onset association disorder* is noted in infants who *normally* awaken frequently, but then receive frequent parental intervention that involves rocking or feeding the infant; the infant then learns to go back to sleep only with "parental assistance," leaving both the infant and parent(s) exhausted from limited normal sleep. Young children may also develop this form of insomnia. *Limit setting sleep disorder* is noted in children 3 years of age and older who develop a refusal to go to bed at a normal time because of lack of regular bedtime encouragement by parents, anxiety, primary sleep disorders, medication effects, or other factors. *Adjustment setting sleep disorder* can occur in children who develop a relatively sudden refusal to go to bed or wake up frequently from sleep, sometimes because of normal nightmares that excessively worry parents, and then the child; the underlying cause is often a traumatic event in the child's life. The therapeutic approach to these three insomnia types is identifying the underlying factors and correcting them with behavioral management.

The older child or adolescent may develop *psychophysiologic insomnia* in which the patient is unable to fall and/or remain asleep due to various factors, such as the development of anxiety about sleep, erratic bedtime schedules, caffeine or other drug effects, underlying medical or psychiatric illnesses, and others. Puberty induces a shift to later bedtimes in many youth partially due to a change in circadian rhythm which may lead to an overt *delayed sleep phase disorder* in which the adolescent goes to bed later and later, while experiencing extreme difficulty getting up in early morning while still in a deep sleep stage. If there is an underlying school avoidant behavior or depression, the child or adolescent may miss much school and be very resistant to correcting this behavior. Management of such delayed sleep onset includes understanding the factors behind the sleep dysfunction and instituting proper behavioral management; medications (as sleeping pills or other medications that induce sedation) only worsen the entire picture and are not recommended. If the child or adolescent develops a significant sleep debt, excessive daytime sleepiness may develop that can result in many episodes of transient, unconscious "microsleeps" that may be misinterpreted as attention span dysfunction.

Sleep dysfunction may result from exposure to high altitude and is termed *altitude insomnia*. There may be abnormal, intermittent breathing (Cheyne–Stokes) noted during non-REM sleep, probably due to effects of both hypocapnia and hypoxia. It typically resolves over a few days as the individual becomes acclimatized to the higher altitude. Severe and/or persistent cases may improve with the use of acetazolamide.

## ■ Excessive daytime sleepiness

Extreme sleepiness during the day, like insomnia at night, is a symptom of underlying issues and not a specific diagnosis. Table 11.7 lists causes of being excessively tired during the day, a condition that can lead to depression, irritability, academic failure, impulsivity, ADHD-like features and even injury and death from motor vehicle accidents.

Children with excessive sleepiness may not actively state they are tired, but may have these same features. As noted earlier, puberty-induced circadian rhythm alternation can lead to young adolescents delaying their bedtime so that they fall asleep in early morning hours and sleep until late morning or early afternoon hours. The development of *delayed sleep phase disorder* (DSPS) can be worsened by *poor sleep hygiene* induced by

**Table 11.7** Causes of excessive daytime sleepiness.

Poor sleep hygiene (see text)

Delayed sleep phase disorder (see text)

Drug effects (as caffeine in caffeinated beverages, alcohol, others; see Table 10.5)

Psychiatric disorders (see Table 10.4)

Medical disorders

• hypothyroidism

• anemia

• infectious mononucleosis

• Lyme disease

• substance abuse disorder

• epilepsy

• central nervous system (CNS) tumor

• trauma to the paramedian thalamic areas of the CNS

Narcolepsy

Klein–Levin syndrome

Restless leg syndrome

Parasomnias

Obstructive sleep apnea/ hypopnea syndrome (OSAHS)

Jet lag (rapid time-zone change) syndrome

Others

the adolescent watching television, listening to music (radio, CD players, MP3 players, etc.), or playing video games in his/her bedroom, having too much light or noise in the bedroom, having a bedroom that is too cold or hot, eating within a few hours of bedtime, consuming any amount of caffeine, and/or several other factors.

Management includes correcting these and other factors that contribute to the specific youth's poor sleep hygiene and behavioral management to correct the abnormal bedtime and awake cycles. The child or adolescent can be exposed to early morning light to help correct the abnormal internal time clock; a light box that provides 2500–10 000 lux for 30 minutes may also help. Exogenous melatonin (1–6 mg at bedtime for 3–6 weeks) has been used to correct circadian rhythm dysfunction, including *rapid time-zone change (jet lag) syndrome*; this latter condition is due to airplane travel through many time zones resulting in daytime sleepiness, insomnia, excessive arousals from sleep, dizziness, and even gastrointestinal symptoms. Sleeping aid medications used to treat insomnia in adults, such as zolpidem (short-acting benzodiazepine receptor agonist) should not be used in children and adolescents. Desperate parents and even adolescents have resorted to sleeping aid measures that are not medically indicated, such as benzodiazepines, chloral hydrate, and over-the-counter cold or cough medications containing alcohol, diphenhydramine, or other sedative ingredients. Chloral hydrate and diphenhydramine have been used at a dose of 25–50 mg, while diazepam has been used at a dose of 0.2 mg/kg shortly before desired bedtime. Use of such sedative medications is not effective and patients may experience tolerance and reactive hyperactive ("wired") behavior as well as other withdrawal effects. Such medications must be tapered even after use for a few days to avoid rebound effects.

## ■ Narcolepsy

Narcolepsy is a well-known primary sleep disorder with an incidence of about 0.1%. It is a chronic neurological disorder characterized by REM sleep dysfunction. A positive family history is noted in 25% of cases, and it may also follow trauma to the CNS. Most patients have some, but not all of the features of narcolepsy: *excessive daytime sleepiness, cataplexy, hypnagogic hallucinations*, and *sleep paralysis*. Some patients have a deficiency of hypocretin, a neuropeptide transmitter involved in the process of staying awake while inhibiting REM sleep. There is an association with two HLA class II antigens: DR2 and DQ1; HLA DQB1*0602 is the most closely associated marker for narcolepsy, particularly for cataplexy. DQA*0102 is also noted with narcolepsy.

*Excessive daytime sleepiness* is associated with REM-onset sleep and typically occurs when the individual is seated or not moving; however, it can be while eating or standing as well. It may be mistaken for causes other than narcolepsy (Table 11.7) and the diagnosis thus delayed for months to years – typically until adulthood. *Cataplexy* is mainly seen in adults in which there is transient loss of tone in striated muscle of the face and extremities; unconsciousness does not occur. Cataplexy can be precipitated by becoming suddenly afraid. *Hypnagogic hallucinations* involve dream-like states that involve various senses and seem very real to the individual; they occur while falling asleep or while waking up. Finally, *sleep paralysis* may occur, in which one cannot move while falling asleep or waking up for a brief time, usually under one minute.

Tables 11.8 lists medications used to treat narcolepsy. Excessive daytime sleepiness is treated with psychostimulant medication (methylphenidate

**Table 11.8** Medications used to manage narcolepsy: daytime sleepiness.

| Class | Agent | Dose | Side effects |
|---|---|---|---|
| Psychostimulants | Methylphenidate (MPH) | 10–60 mg/d; start with 5–10 mg 2×/d; no more than 20 mg in a single dose or 60–80 mg/d; dosing can be a single AM dose or 3×/d. | Both MPH and amphetamines: insomnia, reduced appetite, loss of weight. abdominal pain, headache, depression, rebound symptoms, FDA black box warning on sudden death; tolerance; controlled Schedule II substance with abuse risk; others, see Chapter 4 |
| | Mixed amphetamines Dextroamphetamine Pemoline (rarely used today due to rare adverse effect of liver failure) | Dose similar to MPH dose | |
| Wakefulness promoting agent (long-acting) | Modafinil | Start with 100–200 mg once a day in the morning; some need a morning and noon dose; maximum dose is 400 mg/d. | Not a controlled drug; FDA approved for narcolepsy >14 years of age; headache, nausea, nervousness, rhinitis, diarrhea, back pain, insomnia, dizziness, dyspepsia |

**Table 11.9** Medications used to manage narcolepsy: cataplexy, sleep paralysis, hypnagogic hallucinations.

| Class | Agent | Oral dose | Side effects |
|---|---|---|---|
| SSRIs | Fluoxetine | 10–20 mg/d (up to 60 mg/d) | Insomnia, headache, nausea. See Chapter 5 |
| Other antidepressants | Venlafaxine | 37.5–150 mg/d | Sedation, dry mouth, headache, nausea. See Chapter 5 |
| Tricyclic antidepressants | Imipramine Protriptyline Clomipramine | 50–200 mg/d 10–40 mg/d 25–50 mg/d | Confusion, constipation, dizziness, sedation, dry mouth, tremor, urinary retention, weight gain; see Chapter 5 and Tables 11.10–12 |
| Benzodiazepines | Clonazepam | 0.25 mg–2 mg orally at night. | Adverse effects: sedation, ataxia, confusion; if stopped too soon: rebound reactions. Schedule IV controlled substance |
| Miscellaneous | Sodium oxybate | 6–9 g/d divided in 2 equal doses | FDA-approved for cataplexy; difficult to obtain unless one is a sleep expert; sedation, headache, nausea, dizziness, high abuse potential |

or dextroamphetamine) or modafinil, which is an FDA-approved drug for narcolepsy for those over age 14 years of age and tends to have less adverse effects than the psychostimulants.

Medical management (Table 11.9) of other narcoleptic features (i.e. cataplexy, sleep paralysis, or hypnagogic hallucinations) is with medication that suppresses REM sleep, deep delta sleep, and reduces inter-sleep stage arousals; this includes tricyclic antidepressants, SSRIs, and benzodiazepines (e.g. clonazepam at 0.25–2 mg at night). Cautious use of such medications is recommended, since medication masks and does not directly treat the sleep disorder; caution is also advised since medication leads to such problems as tolerance and rebound when stopping the medication. The result of deep sleep wave suppression while on medication for an extended time is not known at present. Nonpharmacologic management involves attention to proper sleep hygiene along with additional measures for daytime sleepiness, such as use of minimal daytime naps and exercise.

## ■ Klein–Levin syndrome

The Klein–Levin syndrome is a pattern of increased sleeping (up to 20 hours out of 24 hours) associated with periods of confusion, withdrawal, and augmented sexual behavior; it may occur 3–4 times in a year. The hypersomnia may be followed by episodes of bulimia (compulsive overeating), hyperactivity, irritability, hypersexuality (such as excessive masturbation), and even hallucinations. It is mainly described in adolescent males in late puberty, and may be precipitated by serious CNS trauma, viral illness, and stress leading to hypothalamic dysfunction. A sleep study reveals increased REM and non-REM sleep along with short REM latency. The differential diagnosis includes temporal lobe epilepsy, bipolar disorder, and encephalitis. There is no clear research support for the efficacy of stimulant medications; tricyclic antidepressants and anticonvulsant medications have been tried for severe cases. Fortunately, it gradually improves over the course of later adolescence and is usually absent by adulthood.

A variation is called *post-traumatic hypersomnolence* in which prolonged daytime sleepiness and extended nocturnal sleeping develops within a few weeks after severe CNS trauma; the differential diagnosis includes secondary narcolepsy, epilepsy, depression, and encephalopathy. The symptoms may last 6–18 months, usually with full resolution.

## ■ Parasomnias

Parasomnias (Table 11.3) are disorders of arousal (partial or full) and sleep–wake transitioning that involve CNS confusion as well as disturbances of muscle (skeletal and autonomic). Parasomnias are generally more common in children than in adolescents. *Rhythmic movement disorders* involve such movements as body rocking, head rolling, and head banging that start during the first year of life as the infant is at the sleep–wake transition. It can be noted in both normal and developmentally delayed infants, and it resolves before age 4 years. Management involves reassuring the parents of the benign nature of this condition, though bed padding is necessary to protect the infant. Severe cases that continue past infancy, possibly complicated by neuropsychiatric disorders, may respond to the use of benzodiazepines or tricyclic antidepressants.

*Bruxism* or repetitive, nocturnal grinding of teeth is noted in 50% of infants during the period of teeth eruption, though 20% of older children can develop this condition as well, leading to possible temporomandibular joint pain and excessive wearing of dental surfaces. Children with persistent bruxism may benefit from wearing mouth guards at night, analgesics, and biofeedback management; severe cases may respond to judicious use of a benzodiazepine.

*Sleep talking* is a parasomnia that involves seemingly purposeless talking while sleeping; reassurance of the benign nature of this phenomenon is all that is necessary. *Nightmares* develop in the last part of the night when REM sleep is occurring and they can be precipitated by psychological issues including anxiety and sexual abuse; alcohol and other drug withdrawal can also trigger nightmares in adolescents. Management involves reassurance of the benign nature of nightmares and behavioral management for identified triggers.

An example of a partial arousal parasomnia is that of *sleep walking* (or *somnambulism*) in which the individual gets up from sleep and walks, usually in the first part of sleeping at the transition from slow wave Stage 4 sleep. The main principle of management involves reassurance of the benign nature of this condition, unless injury occurs while sleep walking; thus, the house should be safe guarded, alarms set to alert others of the sleep walking, and other protections added for this individual.

Another partial arousal parasomnia is *sleep terrors* (*night terrors* or *pavor nocturnus*) that typically is seen in non-REM sleep and thus not recalled by the patient, who is usually between 4 and 12 years of age. Persistence into adolescence occurs in one-third of cases, and occasionally even into adulthood. The sleep terror begins with vivid vocalizations (i.e. screaming, loud crying) associated with increased heart rate and respirations, as well as sweating. The episode usually does not last over half an hour, but tends to recur at the same time each night. As noted with sleep walking, a genetic predisposition is noted in those with night terrors. If the child or adolescent has underlying factors that prolong slow wave sleep because of sleep deprivation, there may be an increase in night terrors. The differential diagnosis of sleep terrors includes *nocturnal pain attack, complex partial seizure, confusional arousal,* and *temporal lobe epilepsy.* Most situations do not last beyond a year and reassurance is usually all that is necessary. Waking the child or adolescent up within half an hour after falling asleep may help. Correction of underlying factors that can lead to sleep deprivation, such as medications or obstructive sleep apnea, can also be beneficial.

Medication is usually not needed for the partial arousal parasomnias, sleep walking and sleep terrors. Severe or persistent situations may improve with the use of medication that suppresses slow wave sleep or changes the transition from non-REM and REM sleep; these drugs are used for several months (e.g. 3–6) and then stopped to see if the parasomnia resumes. These medications include tricyclic antidepressants (such as imipramine), SSRIs (such as sertraline), or a benzodiazepine (e.g. clonazepam). The latter is given orally at 0.25–2 mg at night; side effects include sedation, confusion, ataxia, and rebound reactions if stopped. Diazepam has been used in adults, but the withdrawal period may be problematic.

Finally, *primary nocturnal enuresis* may be considered a parasomnia as well and refers to bedwetting at night after an age at which nocturnal bladder control is expected, such as 5–7 years of age. The incidence falls from 3% to 4% at age 12 to less than 1% in 19-year-old males. Table 11.10 lists factors associated with primary nocturnal bedwetting. Bedwetting can occur at all sleep stages. Table 11.11 lists causes of secondary enuresis. Behavioral modification is used to manage many cases of primary nocturnal enuresis, including wetting alarms (operant conditioning devices), scheduled voiding programs, counseling, hypnosis, acupuncture, and diet changes. Table 11.12 lists medications used to manage primary nocturnal enuresis.

## ■ Restless legs syndrome (RLS)

This disorder is much better defined in adults than in children or adolescents. Features are discomfort ("crawling-creeping" or aching sensation) in the lower extremities at night (often called "growing pains of childhood") and dysfunctional sleeping patterns, which may begin in childhood; the discomfort is relieved by movement of the affected extremity. Restless legs

**Table 11.10** Factors associated with primary nocturnal bedwetting (NB).

Genetics (75% increased if 2 parents had childhood NB; 45% increase with 1 parent)
Being male
Small bladder
"Heavy sleeper"
Deficiency of nocturnal antidiuretic hormone surge
Chronic illness
Institutionalization
Poverty
Unstable bladder

**Table 11.11** Causes of secondary enuresis.

Diabetes mellitus or insipidus
Posterior water intoxication
Mental subnormality
Hinman–Allen syndrome (non-neurogenic neurogenic bladder)
Unstable bladder
Intake of too much fluid
Consumption of caffeinated beverages
Urinary tract infection
Urethral or bladder obstruction
Lumbosacral abnormality (spinal cord tumor, tethered spinal cord)
Sickle cell disorder (anemia or trait)
Obstructive sleep apnea syndrome (OSAS)
Renal disorders (as tubulointerstitial disease)
Constipation
Anterior labial frenulum displacement
Food allergies

syndrome is often not well described by children or adolescents and often not appreciated by clinicians until the patient "presents" in adulthood with recognized RLS. Children and adolescents may have a delayed onset of sleep because of extremity discomfort, often worse at night and more commonly in lower extremities than the upper. The majority of adults with restless legs syndrome as noted by clinical history have overt *periodic limb movement disorder* (PLMD) that is identified by an overnight sleep study in which periodic foot dorsiflexion and first toe extensions are seen; PLMD is noted in various sleep disorders of adults and may represent a mild peripheral neuropathy in some. Restless legs syndrome may occur in 5% of adults to some extent and one-third of adults have others in their family with this

**Table 11.12** Pharmacologic agents for primary nocturnal enuresis.

| Agent | Dose | Adverse effects | Comments |
|-------|------|-----------------|----------|
| Imipramine | 25–125 mg orally at night | Cholinergic and other tricyclic antidepressant effects: sedation, restlessness, poor concentration, weight loss, syncope, dry mouth (decreased salivary flow and increased tooth decay), blurring of vision (including cycloplegia and mydriasis), confusion, dizziness, constipation, anxiety; urinary retention; drug interactions with SSRIs; EKG changes (sinus tachycardia, AV blocks, increased QRS interval, increased QTc interval); overdose can be fatal with arrhythmias and respiratory depression | Start with 25–50 mg with gradual increase if necessary; 50% will respond; taken 30 minutes before bedtime. If helpful, use for 3–6 months before weaning off. |

| Oxybutynin | 5 mg orally at night; up to 5 mg, 3×/d. Extended release form available for treatment of overactive bladder and also detrussor overactivity due to neurological disorders | Anticholinergic adverse effects including dry mouth, constipation, and flushing; avoid overheating on hot days | Start with low dose and use for 3–6 months if beneficial before gradual weaning off; helps to suppress uninhibited bladder activity; three times daily dose for daytime enuresis seen with unstable bladder. |
|---|---|---|---|
| Desmopressin acetate (synthetic analogue of anti-diuretic hormone [ADH]) | 0.2–0.6 mg orally or 10–40 mcg intranasally at night; one nasal puff is 10 mcg | Anecdotal reports of hyponatremia in those with underlying liver and kidney disease; epistaxis and headaches with the intranasal form | First agent of choice for many clinicians. Start with low dose 20–30 minutes before bedtime; increase after 2–3 weeks to maximum of 3 pills or 4 puffs. The pills can be chewed if necessary. Use the most efficacious dose for 3–6 months before any attempts to wean off. Use with aggressive fluid restriction. |

**Table 11.13** Medications used to treat adults with restless legs syndrome (RLS).

1. Dopamine agonists
   a. Levodopa-carbidopa
   b. Bromocriptine
   c. Pergolide
2. Opioids (Narcotics)
   a. Codeine
   b. Oxycodone
   c. Propoxyphene
3. Anticonvulsants
4. Benzodiazepine
   a. Clonazepam
   b. Diazepam

condition in a partial autosomal dominant pattern. This condition may be worsened by caffeine, increasing sleep debt, diabetic neuropathy, amyloidosis, malignancy, and during pregnancy.

The etiology of RLS is linked to dopaminergic dysfunction and the transient, repetitive lower limb jerks or rhythmic movements occur in sleep Stages 1 and 2 with sleep arousals. There is often a positive family history and also a history that symptoms are worsened with caffeine intake as well as with iron deficiency anemia (as noted by a low ferritin level). Underlying renal failure may also precipitate RLS. Management of RLS involves iron supplementation (if iron deficiency is present) and use of various medications, usually at low doses; medications are mainly used in adults (Table 11.13). Medications used to treat adults with PLMD include dopaminergic drugs and benzodiazepines.

*Ropinirole* is a non-ergoline dopamine agonist approved by the FDA for use in adults with restless legs syndrome. The starting dose for adults is 0.25 mg 1–3 hours before bedtime. The daily dose is then titrated over a period of subsequent 7–8 weeks not to exceed 4 mg per day. It is generally well-tolerated with few side effects. However syncope, bradycardia, and postural hypotension can occur. The product warning indicate that patients may experience sleepiness during activities of daily living that may occur without preceding somnolence or drowsiness. Such falling asleep during day-time activities (including driving) can occur for the first time even after prolonged use.

**Table 11.14** Types of sleep-disordered breathing.

Snoring (with no gas exchange dysfunction)
Upper airway resistance syndrome (UARS)
Obstructive hypoventilation (OH)
Obstructive sleep apnea syndrome (OSAS)

**Table 11.15** Risk factors for obstructive sleep apnea syndrome (OSAS).

Adenotonsillar hypertrophy
Positive family history
Obesity
Craniofacial syndromes
Down syndrome
Asthma
Allergic rhinitis
Prader–Willi syndrome
Cerebral palsy
Ventilatory muscle weakness (due to neuromuscular disorders)
African–American
Chronic sinus disease
Prematurity
Gastroesophageal reflux (GERD)
Micrognathia
Laryngeal web
Laryngomalacia
Laryngeal masses
Arnold–Chiari malformation
Smoke exposure
Mucopolysaccharidoses

# ■ Sleep-disordered breathing

Children and adolescents may present with sleep-disordered breathing due to upper airway obstruction producing a number of conditions (Table 11.14). There is a 2% incidence of obstructive sleep apnea syndrome (OSAS) and obstructive hypoventilation (OH) with an equal male to female ratio in children and adolescents; a 10% incidence for snoring is noted.

Risk factors for OSAS are listed in Table 11.15; the pathophysiology involves increased upper airway resistance because of such issues as

**Table 11.16** Principles of obstructive sleep apnea syndrome (OSAS) management.

1. Rule out disorders noted in Table 11.15
2. Trial of antihistamine medication
3. Trial of protriptyline (REM-suppressant antidepressant)
4. Adenotonsillectomy for enlarged adenoids and tonsils (OSAS, UARS, OH, and select primary snorers)
5. Weight loss measures to treat obesity if present
6. Positive airway pressure to keep airways open while sleeping:
    a. CPAP (continuous positive airway pressure)
    b. B-PAP (bilevel positive airway pressure)
7. Uvulopalatopharyngoplasty (UPPP)
8. Tracheostomy
9. Rapid palatal expansion
10. Supplemental oxygen
11. Medication:
    a. Fluticasone nasal spray: reduce number of obstructions in mild disease
    b. Montelukast for those with obstruction with mild OSA and no allergic rhinitis/atopy

abnormal anatomy as well as abnormal neuromuscular control of the upper airway. There is obstruction to airflow while the child or adolescent breathes at night while sleeping with hypoxemia, hypercarbia (with negative intrathoracic pressure), and paradoxical movement of the chest and abdomen. This leads to snoring, frequent arousals with gasping and choking, sweating, enuresis, and severe sleep dysfunction.

Excessive daytime sleepiness is more common in adults than children or adolescents; however, severe obstruction can lead to daytime sleepiness, growth delay, ventricular hypertrophy, aspiration, gastroesophageal reflux (GERD), hypertension, and increased intracranial pressure. Children and adolescents may have academic dysfunction and failure due to OSAS-induced poor attention span, cognitive dysfunction, poor memory skills, and reduced reaction time. Some are misdiagnosed with ADHD and/or learning disorders. Thus, a careful history and physical examination are necessary along with a sleep diary and an overnight sleep study (polysomnogram) to diagnose OSAS. Allergic rhinitis should be ruled out and a trial of antihistamine medication may be helpful to eliminate allergy as a primary or secondary mechanism. Management principles are outlined in Table 11.16.

**Table 11.17** Non-benzodiazepine hypnotic drugs used in insomnia (Adults).

| Drug and dosage form | Half-life | Use | Daily dosage range (Adult) | Side effects |
|---|---|---|---|---|
| Zolpidem tablet. Immediate release: 5 mg | 2.5 h (immediate release) | Useful in sleep onset and maintenance. Immediate release form is FDA approved for short-term use for insomnia in adults | Immediate release: 5–10 mg before bedtime | Generally well tolerated; in some patients causes excess sedation; can cause dizziness, ataxia, dose-dependent amnesia, hyperexcitability. Tolerance, dependence, and rebound effects uncommon. Sleep architecture generally preserved. Avoid use with other CNS depressants. Overdose can cause respiratory depression. |
| Controlled release: 6.25 mg | | Controlled release may be used for longer periods | Controlled release: 6.25–12.5 mg | |

(cont.)

**Table 11.17** (*Cont.*)

| Drug and dosage form | Half-life | Use | Daily Dosage Range (Adult) | Side effects |
|---|---|---|---|---|
| Zaleplon capsule 5 mg, 10 mg | 1 h | FDA-approved for short-term use in insomnia. Useful in sleep onset and when short duration of sleep is desired (e.g. jet lag) | 10–20 mg before bedtime | As noted above |
| Eszopiclone tablet 1 mg, 2 mg, 3 mg | 6 h | FDA-approved. Can be used long term. Useful in sleep onset and maintenance; reduced nighttime awakenings. Best evidence for long-term safety with no development of tolerance or dependence | 2–3 mg at bedtime | As noted above. Also can cause dry mouth, headache, nervousness, unpleasant taste. Rebound effects very rare |

*Sources:* Stahl SM. 2006. *Essential Psychopharmacology: The Prescriber's Guide.* Cambridge: Cambridge University Press. Thomson Healthcare Inc. 2007. *Physicians' Desk Reference, 61st edn.* Montvale, NJ: Thomson Healthcare, Inc.

# ■ Summary

A variety of sleep disorders in children and adolescents have been reviewed, as listed in Table 11.3. A careful history and physical examination is necessary to identify the cause of sleep dysfunction, often aided with the use of actigraphy and a sleep lab study. *Behavioral management* is the usual recommended treatment for most sleep disorders in children and adolescents, though the judicial use of medications may be helpful for the daytime sleepiness of narcolepsy (psychostimulants and modafinil [Table 11.8]), nonsleepiness aspects of narcolepsy (fluoxetine, venlafaxine, imipramine, protriptyline, clonazepam, others [Table 11.9]), and nocturnal enuresis (imipramine, oxybutynin, and DDAVP).

Other medications are noted that are mainly used in adults with sleep disorders and occasionally in children or adolescents. Nonbenzodiazepines used in adults are listed in Table 11.17.

Another drug used in adult insomnia is *ramelteon*. Ramelteon is a US FDA-approved drug for use in adults with insomnia. It is a melatonin 1 and 2 receptor agonist and belongs to a newer class of drugs called chronohypnotics. Ramelteon is available as an 8 mg tablet. Its half life is 2–5 hours. It lacks any dose response relationship and the effective daily dose can range from 4 mg up to 64 mg. Side effects include dizziness, sedation, fatigue, and headaches. There have been no reports of tolerance, dependence, addiction, or rebound effects. It helps onset of sleep, increases the total duration of sleep, and especially improves circadian rhythm disturbances.

## SELECTED BIBLIOGRAPHY

American Academy of Pediatrics, Subcommittee on Obstructive Sleep Apnea Syndrome, Section on Pediatric Pulmonology. 2002. Clinical practical guidelines: Diagnosis and management of childhood obstructive sleep apnea syndrome. *Pediatrics*, 109:704–12.

American Academy of Sleep Medicine. 2001. *International Classification of Sleep Disorders: Diagnostic and Coding Manual.* Rochester, MN: American Academy of Sleep Medicine.

Blum NJ. 2006. Elimination disorders In Greydanus DE, Patel DR, Pratt HD (Eds.) *Behavioral Pediatrics, 2nd edn.* New York: iUniverse Publishers, pp. 206–35.

Blum NJ, Mason TBA. 2007. Restless legs syndrome: what is a pediatrician to do? *Pediatrics*, 120:438–9.

Espana RA, Scammell TE. 2004. Sleep neurobiology for the clinician. *Sleep*, 27(4):811–20.

Evans JHC. 2001. Evidence-based management of nocturnal enuresis. *Br. Med. J.*, 323:1167–9.

Fallone G, Owens J, Deane J. 2002. Sleepiness in children and adolescents: clinical implications. *Sleep Med. Rev.*, 6(2):287–306.

Fry JM. 1998. Treatment modalities for narcolepsy. *Neurology*, 50(Suppl. 1):S43–8.

Giannotti F, Cortesi F. 2002. Sleep patterns and daytime functions in adolescents: an epidemiological survey of Italian high-school student population. In Carskadon MA (ed.) *Adolescent Sleep Patterns: Biological, Social and Psychological Influences.* New York: Cambridge University Press.

Glazener CM, Evans JH, Peto RE. 2003. Tricyclic and related drugs for nocturnal enuresis in children. *Cochrane Database Syst. Rev.*, 3:CD002117.

Goetting MG, Reijonen J. 2007. Sleep disorders update in children and adolescents. *Prim. Care Clin. Office Pract.*, 34.

Greydanus DE, Torres AD, Wan JH. 2006. Genitourinary and renal disorders. In *Essential Adolescent Medicine*. NY: McGraw-Hill Medical Publishers, pp. 355–9.

Ivanenko A, Tauman R, Gozal D. 2003. Modafinil in the treatment of excessive daytime sleepiness in children. *Sleep Med.*, 4:579–82.

Klackenburg G. 1982. Somnambulism in childhood – prevalence, course, and behavioural correlations. *Acta Pediatr. Scand.*, 71:495–9.

Littner M, Johnson SF, McCall WV *et al.* 2001. Practice parameters for the treatment of narcolepsy: an update for 2000. *Sleep*, 23:451–66.

Makris CM. 2006. Common sleep disorders. In Burg FD, Ingelfinger J, Polin RA, Gershon AA (Eds.) *Current Pediatric Therapy, 18th edn.* Philadelphia, PA: Saunders-Elsevier, pp. 1234–8.

Mindell JA, Owens JA. 2003. *A Clinical Guide to Pediatric Sleep: Diagnosis and Management of Sleep Problems.* Philadelphia, PA: Lippincott Williams & Wilkins.

Owens, JA. 2006. Sleep disorders in children and adolescents. In Greydanus DE, Patel DR, Pratt HD (Eds.) *Behavioral Pediatrics, 2nd Edn.* New York: iUniverse Publishers, 236–64.

Schuen JN. 2006. Sleep disorders in the adolescent. In Greydanus DE, Patel DR, Pratt HD (Eds.) *Essential Adolescent Medicine*. New York: McGraw-Hill Medical Publishers, pp. 281–97.

Spiegel K, Leprout R, Van Cauter E. 1999. Impact of sleep debt on metabolic function. *Lancet*, 354:1435–9.

Walters AS, Mandelbaum DE, Lewin DS, Kugler S, England SJ, Miller M. 2000. Dopaminergic therapy in children with restless legs/periodic limb movements in sleep and ADHD. Dopaminergy Therapy Study Group. *Pediatr. Neurol.*, 22:182–6.

# Tic disorders in children and adolescents

12

## Donald E. Greydanus and Artemis K. Tsitsika

## ■ Definition

Tics are one of the most common neuropsychiatric disturbances in children and adolescents. Tic or habit spasms are movements that are sudden, brief, highly stereotyped, involuntary, and purposeless. Tics are usually listed as motor tics, vocal tics, and, a rare third type, sensory tics. Classification of tic disorders is divided into transient tic disorder, chronic motor/vocal tic disorder and Tourette's syndrome; Table 12.1 lists the DSM–IV–TR definitions of these disorders.

One theory regarding etiology of tics involves central nervous system (CNS) circuitry dysfunction linking various CNS areas, such as the frontal lobe, thalamus, striatum, and globus pallidus. A more recent and controversial theory looks at the potential role of Group A beta-hemolytic streptococcal infection leading to conditions called PANDAS (Pediatric Autoimmune Neuropsychiatric Disorders Associated with Streptococci).

## ■ Epidemiology

Transient tic disorder is noted in 4–20% of children, including young adolescents. There is a 2–3:1 male to female ratio and a positive family history for tics is often present. Voluntary suppression of these tics may occur for minutes to hours, and stress may worsen these tics. There may be eye blinking, shoulder shrugging, facial grimacing and others. Vocal tics are not present and multiple motor tics may occur in uncommon situations. The tics usually disappear spontaneously, often within weeks of their onset.

**Table 12.1** DSM–IV–TR diagnostic criteria for tic disorders.

Transient Tic Disorder
 A. Single or multiple motor and/or vocal tics.
 B. Tics lasting for at least 4 weeks but for no longer than 12 consecutive months.
 C. Age of onset before 18 years.
 D. Tics are not the result of substances such as stimulants or illnesses such as Huntington's disease or post-viral encephalitis.
 E. Criteria for Tourette's syndrome have never been met.

Chronic Motor or Vocal Tic Disorder
 A. Single or multiple motor or vocal tics, but not both, have been present at some time during the illness.
 B. Duration of tics longer than a year without any period longer than 3 months free of tics.
 C. Age of onset before 18 years.
 D. Tics are not the result of substance such as stimulants or illnesses such as Huntington's disease or post-viral encephalitis.
 E. Criteria for Tourette's syndrome have never been met.

Tourette's Disorder
 A. Multiple motor tics and one or more vocal tics.
 B. Duration of tics longer than a year without any period longer than 3 months free of tics.
 C. Age of onset before 18 years.
 D. Tics are not the result of substances such as stimulants or illnesses such as Huntington's disease or post-viral encephalitis.

Tic Disorder Not Otherwise Specified
Presentations that do not meet criteria to be classified as Tourette's syndrome, transient tic disorder or chronic motor or vocal tic disorder. Examples include tics lasting less than 4 weeks, or with age of onset above 18 years or cases with only one motor and one vocal tic.

Reprinted with permission from the *Diagnostic and Statistical Manual of Mental Disorders, Fourth Edition, Text Revision*, (Copyright 2000). Washington, DC: American Psychiatric Association.

Chronic motor tic disorder (chronic tic disorder) is noted in 1–2% of the general population and may be related to Tourette's syndrome; a positive family history is often found and the etiology is related to central nervous system dopamine metabolism dysfunction. Gilles de la Tourette's syndrome (Tourette's syndrome) is noted in 5 per 10 000 and is ten times more common in children versus adults. There is a 3–4:1 male to female ratio and its onset is usually between 2 and 15 years of age; the average age of onset is

**Table 12.2** Involuntary Muscle Movements.[a]

1. **Athetosis**
   Slow, sinuous, writhing, involuntary movement that most frequently involves distal extremities; frequently increased by voluntary movements
2. **Ballismus**
   Wild, flinging, coarse, irregular, involuntary movements beginning in proximal limb muscles.
3. **Chorea**
   Rapid, irregular, nonrepetitive, sudden movement that may involve any muscle or muscle group; these movements generally interfere with voluntary movements.
4. **Dystonia**
   Slow, twisting, involuntary movements associated with changes in muscle tone; movements generally involve trunk and proximal extremity muscles.
5. **Myoclonus**
   Involuntary rapid, shock-like muscular contractions that are generally nonrepetitive; can be increased by voluntary actions.
6. **Spasm**: Slow and prolonged involuntary contraction of a muscle or group of muscles.
7. **Tic**
   Involuntary, repetitive movement of related groups of muscles; movements do not interfere with voluntary muscle movements.
8. **Tremor**
   Involuntary movement that may be a slow or rapid vibration of the involved body part; tremors may get worse with movement (intentional tremor) or may occur only at rest.

---

[a] Used with permission from Kuperman, S. 1992. Tic disorders in children and adolescents. In Greydanus DE, Wolraich ML, (Eds.) *Behavioral Pediatrics*. New York: Springer-Verlag, p. 452.

7 years and, by definition, the end age of onset is age 21. There is often a positive family history for tic disorder, Tourette's syndrome, and/or chronic tic disorder.

# ■ Differential diagnosis/comorbidity

Table 12.2 provides a differential diagnosis of involuntary muscle movements. Tics are not the result of stimulants or illnesses, such as Huntington's disease or post-viral encephalitis. The diagnosis is made in the patient with classic features, as noted in Table 12.1.

**Table 12.3** Tics noted in Tourette's syndrome.

Simple or complex tics involving
  Head
  Neck
  Trunk
  Extremities (upper or lower)

Motor tics
  Eye blinking
  Lip smacking
  Shoulder shrugging
  Head tossing
  Grimacing
  Others

Simple vocal tics
  Coughing
  Grunting
  Shouting
  Crying
  Barking
  Throat clearing
  Sniffing

Complex vocal tics
  Echolalia (repeating words)
  Palilalia (repeating the last sound)
  Coprolalia (swearing)

A wide variety of tics are noted in Tourette's syndrome (Table 12.3). Motor tics usually start before vocal tics and a single tic is the presenting symptom in 50%; multiple tics are also seen in 50% of patients. The presenting tic is the eye tic in 37%, the head tic in 16%, and a vocal tic in 18%. Coprolalia is the presenting feature in 0.1%, though one-third of patients with Tourette's syndrome eventually develop this classic swearing feature. A sensory tic is noted in 3% in which an unpleasant sensation develops about a joint or muscle group that is relieved with a motor tic. Voluntary suppression of tics is characteristic for a brief period of time; however, a feeling of unpleasantness develops, leading to the tic.

Table 12.4 lists conditions associated with Tourette's syndrome. For example, Attention deficit/hyperactivity disorder is noted in 30–50% of children

**Table 12.4** Conditions associated with tourette's syndrome.

| Condition | Frequency (estimated %) |
|---|---|
| Attention-deficit/hyperactivity disorder | 50–60 |
| Obsessive–compulsive disorder | 25–50 |
| Other anxiety disorders | 30–40 |
| Mood disorders | 30–40 |
| Learning disorders (± ADHD) | 20–30 |
| Disruptive behavior disorders | Common, but more related to ADHD |
| Explosive anger ("rage"), including intermittent explosive disorder | Common, related to ADHD and mood disorders |
| Substance-use disorders | Unknown, but increases with age |
| Pervasive developmental disorders | Unknown, but likely low |

and adolescents with Tourette's syndrome; Obsessive–compulsive disorder is found in 30–60%. Patient education about Tourette's syndrome can be obtained at the web site of the Tourette's syndrome Association from the USA at http://www.tsa-usa.org.

# ■ Psychopharmacology

Tic disorders often require a wide range of treatment from education of the patient to intensive behavioral therapy to actual use of psychotropic medications. Transient tic disorder often disappears spontaneously within one year, often within several weeks. Thus, specific medical management is usually not necessary, unless tic progression develops in unusual situations. Chronic motor tic disorder and Tourette's syndrome typically require the use of psychopharmacologic agents (Table 12.5) that traditionally have included haloperidol, pimozide, and clonidine. A variety of other medications have been used to ameliorate tics, but with less anecdotal and research support.

Most of the medications listed in Table 12.5 are followed by the empirical research designation letters A, B, or C. Category A denotes good supportive evidence for efficacy and safety (based on ≥ 2 randomized, placebo-controlled studies); Category B denotes fair supportive evidence (based on a minimum of one placebo-controlled study); and Category C represents minimal supportive evidence, based on less rigorous sources (such as open-label studies, case reports, etc.).

**Table 12.5** Medications used in persons with Tourette's syndrome and comorbid disorders, and ages at which use may be appropriate.

| Class | Agent (A–C)[a] | Doses[b] | Ages[c] |
|---|---|---|---|
| Antipsychotics | | | |
| *First-generation* | | | |
| Phenothiazines | Fluphenazine (B) | 1.5–10 mg/d | ≥18 |
| Butyrophenones | Haloperidol (A) | 1–4 mg/d | ≥18; ≥3[d] |
| Other | Pimozide (A) | 0.05–0.2 mg/kg/d | ≥12 |
| *Second-generation* | Risperidone (A) | 0.25–2 mg, 1–2×/d | ≥18 |
| | Ziprasidone (B) | 5–40 mg/d | ≥18 |
| | Olanzapine (C) | 2.5–12.5 mg/d | ≥18 |
| | Quetiapine (C) | 25–150 mg/d | ≥18 |
| *Partial DA agonist* | Aripiprazole (C) | 10–20 mg/d | ≥18 |
| Alpha-agonists | Clonidine (B) | 0.05–0.3 mg/d | ≥12 |
| | Guanfacine (B) | 0.5–1 mg, 3×/d | ≥12 |
| Anticonvulsants | Topiramate | 50–200 mg/d | ≥2 |
| | Levetiracetam | 1–2 g/d | ≥16 |
| Antidepressants | | | |
| SSRIs (for OCD) | Fluoxetine (A) | 10–60 mg/d | ≥7 |
| | Sertraline (A) | 50–250 mg/d | ≥6 |
| | Fluvoxamine (A) | 50–350 mg/d | ≥6 |
| | Paroxetine (B) | 10–60 mg/d | ≥18 |
| | Citalopram (B) | 20–60 mg/d | N/A |
| | Escitalopram (B) | 10–20 mg/d | N/A |
| Other (for ADHD) | Atomoxetine | 0.5–1.2 mg/kg/d | ≥6 |
| DA receptor agonists | Pergolide (B) | 0.1–0.4 mg/d | ≥18 |
| Muscle relaxants | Baclofen (C) | 5–20 mg, 3×/d | ≥12 |
| Miscellaneous | Nicotine patch (C) | 7–21 mg/d | ≥18 |
| | Mecamylamine (C) | 2.5–7.5 mg/d | ≥18 |
| | Tetrabenazine (C) | 12.5–25 mg, 1–3×/d | ≥18 |

Psychostimulants: See Chapter 5 for details

[a] Empirical support categories (see "Psychopharmacology" for a description).
[b] Dosing is clinically-based, unless stated otherwise.
[c] Ages (years) are for FDA-approved indications (see Table 3.1, Chapter 3, for details); use for other indications and/or at other ages is based on clinical judgement.
[d] For "severe behavioral problems." DA, Dopamine.

# Medication classification and mechanism of action

## Antipsychotics

It is unclear exactly how the antipsychotics work in reducing the tics of Tourette's syndrome and other tic disorders. However, it is presumed that a major part of the mechanism involves dopamine blockade of postsynaptic receptors somewhere in the cortico-striato-thalamic-cortical circuitry.

## Alpha agonists

Alpha agonists help to reduce adrenergic outflow from the CNS; how this lowers tic activity is uncertain.

## Dopamine receptor agonists

The use of dopamine receptor agonists to treat Tourette's syndrome seems counterintuitive, given that the effective antipsychotic agents are dopamine antagonists. These medications, at low doses, do seem to reduce the frequency of tic activity. The hypothesized mechanism of action involves agonism at presynaptic dopamine receptors.

## Muscle relaxants

The benzodiazepines can reduce tic severity in patients, but they are less effective than the antipsychotics. Baclofen may also be helpful, and may involve inhibition via gamma-aminobutyric acid (GABA, of which baclofen is an analog).

## Stimulants

These medications increase availability of dopamine and norepinephrine at postsynaptic neurons, likely via reuptake blockade, or increased release, at presynaptic neurons.

## Antidepressants

These medications exert their effects by increasing catecholamine availability via reuptake inhibition, presynaptic antagonism, postsynaptic antagonism, or a combination of mechanisms. The most commonly used antidepressants in patients with Tourette's syndrome are the selective serotonin reuptake inhibitors, or SSRIs.

## Anticonvulsants

Hypothesized mechanisms of action of anticonvulsants include neuronal membrane stabilization, the inhibition of excitatory amino acids (e.g. glutamate and aspartate), and the increase of GABA, a known inhibitory neurotransmitter.

## Others

Nicotine receptor agonism (via a nicotine patch) and antagonism (with mecamylamine) have shown limited success in reducing the symptoms of Tourette's syndrome; further study is anticipated. Tetrabenazine has two main mechanisms of action; one is depletion of catecholamines from presynaptic neurons, the other is postsynaptic dopamine antagonism.

## Dosages

The dosage ranges listed in Table 12.5 are recommended averages. The amount of starting medication should be adjusted to fit the age, weight, medical status, and symptom severity of the patient.

## Antipsychotics

For haloperidol, one should start with 0.25 mg each day, and increase to 2 mg, two times per day orally, as tolerated. Although higher doses may be used (e.g. 5 mg twice daily), tics generally respond to doses lower than those used to treat psychosis (see Chapter 8).

For pimozide, starting with 1 mg daily and increasing up to 4 mg two times per day is one approach. A safer strategy may be to dose by weight, 0.05–0.2 mg/kg/day, with dosing not to exceed 10 mg daily.

Dosing for risperidone is similar to that of haloperidol.

## Alpha agonists

Clonidine is a presynaptic, central-acting alpha$_2$ adrenergic agonist that is used to improve tic symptoms. Its daily dose range is 0.05–0.3 mg/day; depending on its use, clonidine is provided 2–4 times a day or only at bedtime.

Guanfacine is an alpha$_{2A}$ adrenergic agonist related to clonidine, and is also used to reduce tic frequency. Its daily dosage range is 0.5–1 mg, three times a day.

## Dopamine receptor agonists

Pergolide is used cautiously, starting at 0.1 mg daily, with a gradual increase to a maximum of 0.4 mg daily.

## Muscle relaxants

Baclofen is started at 5 mg, 3 times daily, with increases every 5 days, as needed, to a maximum of 20 mg, 3 times daily (lower than the 80 mg/day maximum in adults).

## Stimulants

Attention deficit/hyperactivity disorder is found in 50% or more of patients with Tourette's syndrome. Children and adolescents with both ADHD and Tourette's may be given both stimulant medications (if effective) and anti-tic medications (such as pimozide or haloperidol) if tics develop. Research does not suggest that stimulant medications cause Tourette's; however, these medications should be used in a "start low and go slow" manner (see Chapter 4 for details on dosing).

## Antidepressants

The SSRIs have been used to improve various comorbidities of Tourette's syndrome, such as phobias, obsessive–compulsive disorder, and generalized anxiety disorder (Table 12.4). Anxiety may worsen tics and thus, anxiety reduction may lead to tic reduction as well (see Chapter 4 for more on the treatment of anxiety disorders; see Chapter 6 for more on the antidepressants).

## Anticonvulsants

There are few data to guide dosing of the anticonvulsants topiramate and levetiracetam to treat Tourette's syndrome. However, topiramate has been used at oral doses ranging from 50–200 mg once per day and levetiracetam has been used at 1000–2000 mg once per day.

## Others

Nicotine patches are available without prescription in the USA. They come in dosages of 7, 14, and 21 mg/patch. The lowest effective dose should be used. Mecamylamine is started at 2.5 mg daily, with a maximum of 2.5 mg, 3 times daily. The time between dosage increases should probably be longer than the 2 days recommended for adults. Tetrabenazine is started with one-half of a 25 mg tablet daily, and titrated by 12.5 mg weekly; maximum dosage in children would likely not exceed 75 mg daily.

## Side effects/adverse effects
### Antipsychotics (see Chapter 8)
The antipsychotics haloperidol, pimozide, and risperidone are the most effective at treating the tics of Tourette's syndrome. They are also the most likely to cause extrapyramidal symptoms (EPS) and neuroleptic malignant syndrome (NMS). Pimozide can also prolong the $QT_c$ interval. The atypical antipsychotics (AA) risperidone, quetiapine, and olanzapine (in increasing order) tend to cause weight gain, and all of the AA can elevate blood glucose to varying degrees. With the exception of quetiapine and aripiprazole, the newer antipsychotics used in Tourette's syndrome can elevate serum prolactin.

### Alpha agonists
Common side effects include dry mouth, drowsiness, dizziness, constipation, and sedation. Children may experience orthostatic hypotension, but it is uncommon. Children may be more susceptible to the rebound hypertension associated with the abrupt discontinuation of the alpha agonist.

### Dopamine receptor agonists
The most common side effects with pergolide refer to the nervous system. Other frequently experienced side effects include gastrointestinal upset, dry mouth, anemia, weight changes, dyspnea, cough, sweating, diplopia, and urinary frequency.

### Muscle relaxants
Baclofen produces a transient somnolence in over half of the patients who take it. Other common side effects include dizziness, weakness, fatigue, confusion, headache, nausea, and urinary frequency. In a few patients receiving baclofen, laboratory testing has disclosed increased SGOT, alkaline phosphatase, and blood sugar.

## Stimulants (see Chapter 5)

These medications can cause stomach upset, decreased appetite, psychomotor agitation, irritability, and insomnia, even if given early in the day.

## Antidepressants

The SSRIs commonly cause stomach upset and nausea, diarrhea, and insomnia. They can also activate patients to the point of agitation, and even akathisia. In susceptible individuals they can destabilize mood, leading to anger and aggression, and even causing mania.

## Anticonvulsants

Topiramate can produce sedation, fatigue, cognitive slowing, behavioral changes, word finding difficulty, precipitation of glaucoma, anemia, dehydration, and renal stones. Levetiracetam's most common side effects include weakness, headache, dizziness, and somnolence. Anticonvulsants may increase risk for suicidality (FDA, 2008).

## Others

Acute adverse effects from nicotine are increases in pulse rate, blood pressure, psychomotor activity, headache, and nausea. The concern for longer-term use is addiction to the nicotine. Mecamylamine may cause constipation (and occasionally ileus), orthostatic hypotension, seizures, abnormal movements, urinary retention, blurred vision, weakness, fatigue, and sedation. Tetrabenazine may cause drowsiness, nervousness, anxiety, restlessness, insomnia, parkinsonism, akathisia, and depression.

# Contraindications

## Antipsychotics

Haloperidol and fluphenazine are contraindicated in patients with blood dyscrasias, hepatic disease, subcortical brain damage, and mental obtundation.

Pimozide should not be used in tic disorders other than Tourette's syndrome. Concurrent use with stimulant medications is discouraged if there is suspicion that the stimulant, and not Tourette's, is the cause of the tics. Pimozide should not be used with any other medications that may combine to prolong the QTc interval, including the psychotropics thioridazine, chlorpromazine, nefazodone, fluvoxamine, fluoxetine, sertraline, ziprasidone, and citalopram.

## Alpha agonists
There are no known specific contraindications to the use of alpha agonists.

## Dopamine receptor agonists
Pergolide should not be used in patients who are hypersensitive to this drug or other ergot derivatives.

## Muscle relaxants
There is no specific contraindication to the use of baclofen.

## Stimulants
These medications should probably be avoided in patients who are already experiencing significant levels of anxiety, tension, or psychomotor agitation. Stimulants should not be used if glaucoma is present. The use of the mixed amphetamines is contraindicated if the patient has symptomatic cardiovascular disease, hypertension, or hyperthyroidism. Their use in patients with Tourette's should be approached with caution. A relative contraindication also exists in the presence of a seizure disorder.

## Antidepressants
All antidepressants with serotonergic activity (except mirtazapine and venlafaxine) are contraindicated for use with pimozide, the combination of which can greatly prolong the $QT_c$ interval.

## Anticonvulsants
There are no specific contraindications to the use of topiramate or levetiracetam.

## Others
Both nicotine and mecamylamine are contraindicated in patients with hypertension. Mecamylamine should also not be used if the patient has renal insufficiency, glaucoma, or is taking antibiotics. Tetrabenazine may

cause a recurrence or exacerbation of depression in patients with a prior or current episode, respectively, of depression.

## How to use the medications

### Antipsychotics

If tics are severe and/or bothersome to the patient, and they have not responded to the alpha agonists (see below) and/or behavioral interventions, a trial of an antipsychotic is warranted. Even with aggressive treatment, complete tic suppression may not be possible, thus reduction in tic frequency may be the management goal along with education about the tic disorder itself.

Two common medications which have traditionally been used for tic suppression are haloperidol and pimozide, but risperidone has become more popular of late. No matter which agent is chosen, a general rule in using these agents in children and adolescents is to start with a low dose and titrate slowly upwards to seek the best balance between tic amelioration and minimization of adverse effects.

Approximately one fourth of patients placed on haloperidol experience a 70% reduction in tics at a dose that avoids major side effects; 50% note a reduction in tics only at a dose that leads to major side effects, and 25% do not respond to haloperidol. Pimozide can lead to a 70–80% reduction in tics, often without development of serious side effects. Risperidone has been used to suppress tics at an oral dose that ranges from 0.25 mg a day to 2 mg twice a day.

### Alpha agonists

These medications are suggested as the first-line agents when pharmacotherapy is needed to treat the tics of Tourette's syndrome. Clonidine is also used as an alternative or adjunctive medication to stimulants for ADHD, and to help with post-traumatic stress disorder, and severe aggressiveness with conduct disorder or oppositional defiant disorder (see Chapters 5 and 7). Gradual build-up and withdrawal when using clonidine are recommended; rapid withdrawal may lead to rebound hypertension. Sedation is a major limiting factor in using this medication.

Guanfacine use may result in less blood pressure problems and sedation than seen with clonidine. Adverse reactions are similar to clonidine, but there may be more agitation and headaches, so patients should be monitored closely.

## Dopamine receptor agonists

As the use of this medication in Tourette's is experimental, extreme caution should be taken when used in children and adolescents. Pergolide may cause somnolence and the possibility of falling asleep during activities of daily living; therefore, patients should be cautioned about certain activities (e.g. bike riding, skateboarding, roller skating) until there is reasonable certainty that the medication does not affect them adversely. Caution should be used when patients are taking other CNS depressants in combination with pergolide.

## Muscle relaxants

The clinical approach to use of baclofen – and the associated cautions – are similar to those of pergolide.

## Stimulants

If the tics are worsened by the stimulant drugs, other anti-ADHD medications may be tried that do not typically worsen tics; these include alpha$_2$ agonists (such as clonidine or guanfacine) or atomoxetine, a selective norepinephrine reuptake inhibitor (Chapter 4). Atomoxetine is given at an oral dose ranging from 0.5–1.2 mg/kg per day. The US FDA has given atomoxetine a black box warning due to a rare adverse effect of severe liver toxicity. The antidepressant bupropion may improve the symptoms of ADHD, but may also worsen tics.

## Antidepressants

Table 12.5 lists the SSRIs that have been used to improve the symptoms of obsessive–compulsive disorder associated with Tourette's syndrome. Of the listed agents, citalopram and escitalopram are less likely to lead to behavioral activation and agitation; thus, their use is preferred by some experts. No matter which antidepressant is used for obsessive–compulsive disorder, there is a tendency for successful treatment to require high doses, sometimes above the range recommended for the treatment of depression. Close monitoring is necessary to prevent or minimize medication side effects.

## Anticonvulsants

The use of topiramate and levetiracetam is strictly clinical, so the previous caution of "start low and go slow" applies to these agents as well. This is especially relevant in the presence of renal impairment.

## Others

The use of the nicotine patch is guided by clinical response and tolerance. It should be applied in the morning and taken off in the late afternoon or early evening. Mecamylamine absorption improves when taken with food, and sedation can be better tolerated if it is given later in the day. Tetrabenazine is absorbed unevenly after oral dosing. It should therefore be taken 2–3 times daily for greatest effect. This medication is not sold in the USA, but can be purchased legally from Canada (with a valid prescription), as the FDA has classified tetrabenazine as an orphan drug, with fast-track status.

## How to monitor the medications

### Antipsychotics

The patient's height, weight, and BMI (body–mass index) should be measured before starting antipsychotic medications and at each subsequent visit. Blood pressure and pulse should be checked at baseline, and then at least every 3 months. Fasting glucose and lipids should be measured before starting treatment, after 3 months, and then every 6 months thereafter. A baseline examination for extrapyramidal signs should be recorded, and re-checked during dosage escalations, and then once every 3 months. The use of the pimozide or ziprasidone requires baseline and follow-up ECGs, particularly during dosage titrations. Prolactin should be checked at any point if menstrual or sexual problems develop.

### Alpha agonists

When prescribing clonidine, take some baseline data (blood pressure, pulse, blood sugar, ECG); follow these data on a regular basis, including a repeat ECG every 6 months. A few cardiac-related deaths have been reported in children and adolescents taking both methylphenidate and clonidine simultaneously. No specific laboratory testing is required.

### Dopamine receptor agonists

No specific laboratory tests are necessary for the management of patients on pergolide. Periodic routine evaluation of all patients should be carried out at appropriate times. Blood pressure and pulse should be checked at home and during clinical visits.

### Muscle relaxants

For patients on baclofen, periodic laboratory testing for SGOT, alkaline phosphatase, and blood sugar should be ordered.

### Stimulants

During chronic treatment with these agents, periodic complete blood count (CBC), with differential and platelet count, is recommended. Blood pressure and pulse should be checked at each medication visit. Height and weight should be measured per routine schedule, and any significant slowing, stoppage, or loss should prompt discontinuation and medical evaluation.

### Antidepressants

No routine laboratory tests are required for any of the SSRIs.

### Anticonvulsants

Patients on topiramate should have a periodic CBC, and BUN and creatinine. The medication infrequently causes increases of liver function tests. No routine laboratory tests are recommended for patients on levetiracetam.

### Others

For patients on the nicotine patch or mecamylamine, blood pressure and pulse should be checked routinely at home and during clinical visits. Patients treated with tetrabenazine should be screened at each visit for symptoms of depression.

## ■ Summary

The safe and effective treatment of Tourette's disorder, and other tic disorders, is based on a logical hierarchy of interventions, from cognitive and behavioral therapies to pharmacologic agents. Figure 12.1 illustrates one example of a treatment algorithm; other approaches may be found in the medical literature.

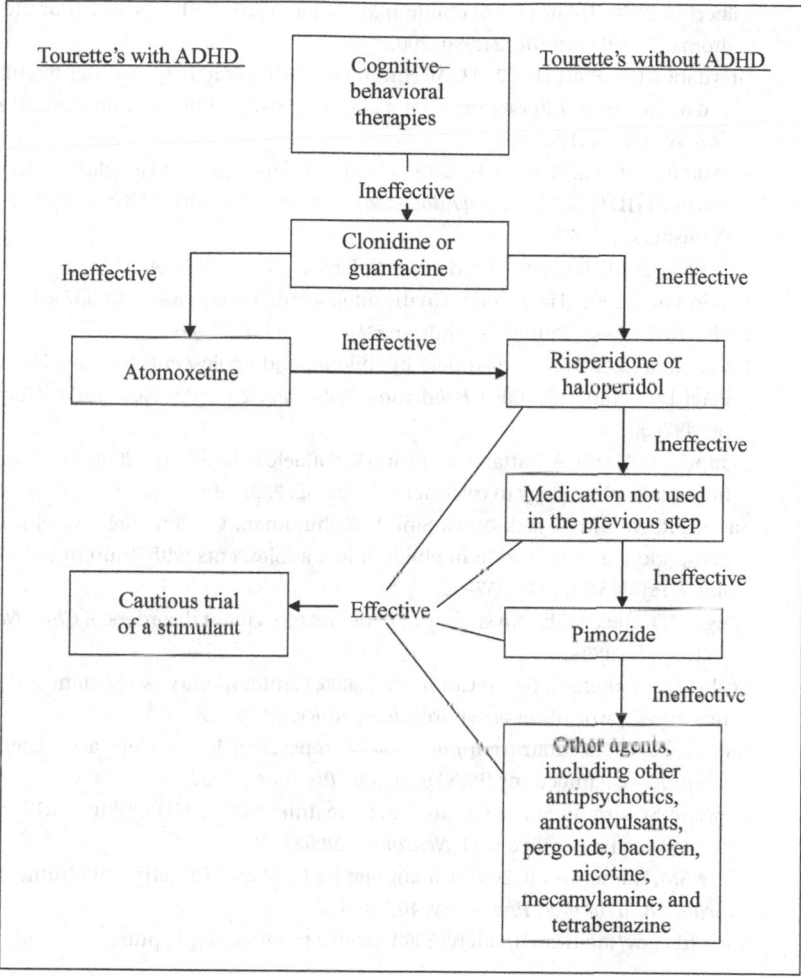

**Figure 12.1** Treatment algorithm for Tourette's syndrome, with/without ADHD.

## SELECTED BIBLIOGRAPHY

Cohen DJ, Young JG, Nathanson JA, Shaywitz BA. 1979. Clonidine in Tourette's syndrome. *Lancet*, 2:551–3.

Delgado MR, Albright AL. 2003. Movement disorders in children: definitions, classifications and grading systems. *J. Child Neurol.* 18 (Suppl. 1):S1–8.

Edgar, TS. 2003. Oral pharmacotherapy of childhood movement disorders. *J. Child Neurol.* 18 (Suppl. 1):S40–9.

Gaffney GR, Perry PJ, Lund BC, Bever-Stiller KA, Arndt S, Kuperman S. 2002. Risperidone versus clonidine in the treatment of children and adolescents with Tourette's syndrome. *J. Am. Acad. Child Adolesc. Psychiatry*, 41:330–6.

Gilbert D. 2006. Treatment of children and adolescents with tics and Tourette syndrome. *J. Child Neurol.*, 21:690–700.

Greydanus DE, Pratt HD. 2003. Attention-deficit/hyperactivity disorder in children and adolescents: Interventions for a complex costly clinical conundrum. *Pediatr. Clin. N. Am.*, 50:1049–92.

Greydanus DE, Van Dyke DH. 2006. Neurologic disorders. In Greydanus DE, Patel DR, Pratt HD (Eds.) *Essential Adolescent Medicine.* New York: McGraw-Hill Medical Publishers, 235–79.

Jankovic J. 2001. Tourette's syndrome. *N. Engl. J. Med.*, 345:1184–92.

Kuperman S. 2002. Tic disorders in the adolescent. *Adolesc. Med.*, 13:537–51.

Leckman JF. 2002. Tourette's syndrome. *Lancet*, 360:1577–86.

Pina-Garza JE. 2006. Tic disorders in children and adolescents. In Greydanus DE, Patel DR, Pratt HD (Eds.) *Behavioral Pediatrics*, 2nd edn. New York: iUniverse, pp. 497–507.

Rampello L, Alvano A, Battaglia G, Bruno V, Raffaele R, Nicoletti F. 2006. Tic disorders: from pathophysiology to treatment. *J. Neurol.*, 253:1–15.

Sallee FR, Nesbitt L, Jackson C, Sine L, Sethuraman, G. 1997. Relative efficacy of haloperidol and pimozide in children and adolescents with Tourette's disorder. *Am. J. Psychiatry*, 154:1057–62.

Sanger TD. 2003. Pathophysiology of pediatric movement disorders. *J. Child Neurol.* 18 (Suppl. 1):S9–24.

Scahill L, Erenberg G, Berlin CM Jr *et al.* 2006. Contemporary assessment and pharmacotherapy of Tourette syndrome. *NeuroRx*, 3:192–206.

Swedo SE. 2002. Pediatric autoimmune neuropsychiatric disorders: associated with streptococcal infections (PANDAS). *Mol. Psychiatry*, 7:S24–5.

Tourette Syndrome Study Group. 2002. Treatment of ADHD children with tics: a randomized controlled trial. *Neurology*, 58:527–36.

Wehr AM, Namerow LB. 2001. Citalopram for OCD and Tourette's syndrome. *J. Am. Acad. Child Adolesc. Psychiatry*, 40:740–1.

www.fda.gov/medwatch/safety/2008/safety08.htm#Antiepileptic

# Substance abuse disorders

## 13

## ■ Introduction

Substance abuse is a major public health conundrum of adolescents and adults throughout the world. The major problem of addiction in the world has intensified since the unfortunate biochemical isolation of cocaine, heroin, and morphine in the nineteenth century. Criteria for substance abuse disorders are often based on definitions of the American Psychiatric Association's *Diagnostic and Statistical Manual of Mental Disorders, Fourth Edition, Text Revision* (DSM–IV–TR) that reflect a number of key symptoms. These definitions, however, are based on adult models, and not adolescents with various degrees of substance use and abuse patterns. DSM–IV–TR views substance abuse as a mental disorder that involves use of drugs or alcohol to the point that major life dysfunction occurs. Substance dependence involves at least three of seven DSM–IV–TR criteria as listed in Table 13.1.

Table 13.2 lists drugs of abuse and Table 13.3 reviews the use of selected illicit drugs by American adolescents from 2001 to 2005.

The epidemiology of adolescent substance abuse in selected European countries is summarized in Figure 13.1.

Prevalence rates for substance abuse or dependence range from 3–4% in middle adolescents to 10% in older youth (ages 17–19 years). Among patients admitted for substance abuse disorders, an increasing number report they started their drug use before age 13. Adolescents who have substance abuse disorders have increased risk for suicide, motor vehicle accidents, and hospitalizations due to drug overdose. As many as 3 out of 4 youth with a substance abuse disorder also have other mental health disorders (Table 13.4).

**Table 13.1** DSM–IV–TR criteria for substance dependence (three or more).

1. Tolerance (need for increased amounts of drug for same desired effect)
2. Withdrawal (symptoms that result from cessation of the drug)
3. Consuming a greater amount of the drug than intended (or intended time)
4. Failed attempts to stop/control drug use or persistent desire for the drug
5. Continued drug use despite knowledge of the drug's negative effects
6. Excess of time spent in pursuing the drug or getting over its effects
7. Chaotic life: less time in school, work, or other important aspects of life

DSM–IV–TR: *Diagnostic and Statistical Manual of Mental Disorders*, Fourth Edn, *Text Revision, 2000.*

**Table 13.2** Drugs of abuse.

Alcohol
Tobacco
Marijuana
Amphetamine
Methamphetamine
Heroin
Cocaine
Hallucinogens
   LSD [lysergic acid diethylamide]
   PCP [phencyclidine]
Date rape drugs
   MDMA ["Ecstasy"]
   Flunitrazepam [Rohypnol]
   Gamma-hydroxybutyrate [GHB]
   Ketamine [Ketalar]
Inhalant drugs
Barbiturates

Research over the past decade has noted that addiction is not an illness that is simply inherited, but a complex illness in which various genes combine with each addict's environment that includes influences of peers and family. Addiction is a chronic disorder that involves using drugs that provide euphoric effects in diverse ways, including enhancing the neurotransmitter *dopamine* in the areas of the brain involved in reward and motivation – such as the mesocorticolimbic pathway.

An important goal of the US Government's Centers for Disease Control and Prevention's Healthy People 2010 is reduced substance use by children and adolescents. The key to reducing the burden that illicit drugs have

**Table 13.3** Percentage of adolescents reporting past-month illicit drug use.[a]

| Year | Percentage (%) |
|------|----------------|
| 2001 | 19.4 |
| 2002 | 18.2 |
| 2003 | 17.3 |
| 2004 | 16.1 |
| 2005 | 15.8 |

[a] Combined data of 50 000 students (8th, 10th, and 12th graders) in USA. From 2005 *Monitoring the Future Study*, the University of Michigan (Lloyd Johnston).

placed on children and adolescents is in *preventing* the drug use and abuse in the first place. Protective factors for substance abuse are considered in Table 13.5, while substance abuse risk factors are listed in Table 13.6; non-specific markers for substance abuse are noted in Table 13.7.

The role of pharmacologic agents in the management of substance abuse disorders in adolescents is secondary or adjunctive, with psychological therapies serving as the primary methods of treatment. Medications may serve a more primary role in the transient issue of helping in acute management of drug intoxication or withdrawal states. Nonpharmacologic management of substance abuse disorders in adolescents include motivational interviewing, cognitive–behavioral therapy, behavior motivation therapy, family therapy, and group counseling. Adolescents may require outpatient treatment, partial hospitalization, inpatient management, detoxification management, acute residential management, and even management in long-term residential programs.

This chapter discusses *alcohol, tobacco, marijuana, hallucinogens, heroin, cocaine*, and other illicit drugs, including *date rape drugs*. The literature on psychopharmacologic management of drug abuse mainly focuses on adults, and there are no medications that are FDA-approved for those with drug abuse under 18 years of age. Many of these medications, however, are used by various clinicians dealing with adolescents who have drug withdrawal and dependence problems.

*Inhalant drugs* include such chemicals as paint thinners or solvents, gasoline, airplane glue, art or office supply solvents, gases (from butane

| Country | Cigarette Smoking | Alcohol Consumption | Cannabis | Lifetime use of other illicit drugs | | | |
|---|---|---|---|---|---|---|---|
| | Lifetime use ≥40 times | Lifetime use ≥40 times | Lifetime | Amphetamines | LSD | Ecstasy | Inhalants |
| *Bulgaria* | 36 | 16 | 12 | 1 | 1 | 1 | 3 |
| *Croatia* | 28 | 18 | 16 | 2 | 2 | 3 | 13 |
| *Czech Republic* | 36 | 41 | 35 | 5 | 5 | 4 | 7 |
| *Denmark* | 32 | 59 | 24 | 4 | 1 | 3 | 7 |
| *Estonia* | 27 | 21 | 13 | 7 | 2 | 3 | 7 |
| *France* | .. | 20 | 35 | 2 | 1 | 3 | 11 |
| *Greece* | 27 | 42 | 9 | 1 | 2 | 2 | 14 |
| *Hungary* | 28 | 13 | 11 | 2 | 3 | 3 | 4 |
| *Ireland* | 34 | 40 | 32 | 3 | 5 | 5 | 22 |
| *Italy* | 25 | 17 | 25 | 2 | 2 | 2 | 6 |
| *Poland* | 26 | 26 | 14 | 7 | 4 | 3 | 9 |
| *Portugal* | 17 | 15 | 8 | 3 | 1 | 2 | 3 |
| *Romania* | 16 | 18 | 1 | 0 | 0 | 0 | 1 |
| *Slovak Republic* | 30 | 27 | 19 | 1 | 3 | 2 | 7 |
| *Slovenia* | 26 | 23 | 25 | 1 | 2 | 4 | 14 |
| *United Kingdom* | 26 | 47 | 35 | 8 | 5 | 3 | 15 |
| *The Netherlands* | 30 | 37 | 28 | 2 | .. | 4 | .. |

**Figure 13.1** Epidemiology of substance abuse in Europe. From The 1999 ESPAD (The European School Survey Project on Alcohol and Other Drugs) Report.

**Table 13.4** Disorders comorbid with substance abuse disorders.

- Attention deficit/hyperactivity disorder
- Anxiety disorders
- Conduct disorder
- Mood disorders
- Oppositional defiant disorder
- Post-traumatic stress disorder
- Psychosis

**Table 13.5** Factors protective of substance abuse in adolescents.

- Academic success in supportive schools of academic excellence
- Adult role models who are supportive and positive
- Adult supervision that is appropriate
- Appropriate assertiveness
- Good social skills
- Good intelligence that allows success in school
- Healthy family communication with loving parents
- Lack of poor health
- Nurturing home environment
- Religiosity and a good moral sense
- Self-esteem that is uplifting and positive
- Supportive peer group who follow healthy lifestyles

lighters, whipping cream aerosols, deodorant sprays, others), ether, chloroform, amyl nitrite or butyl nitrite ("poppers"), and others. These drugs are popular with young adolescents, as there is ready availability. What will not be reviewed in this chapter are drugs used in attempts to improve sports performance (sports doping), such as anabolic steroids.

# ■ Specific drugs of abuse

## Alcohol

Alcohol is among the most abused chemicals in the world because of its widespread acceptance by adolescents and adults. Alcohol consumption is widely encouraged by advertisements in various media, such as movies, magazines, television, and others. Over 85 000 annual deaths are due to excessive alcohol use in the USA, making alcohol the third leading preventable cause of death. In the USA, alcohol is first tried on average at age 12 years, and 17- to 18-year-old youth who are in school have a lifetime

**Table 13.6** Risk factors for substance abuse in adolescents.[a]

| | | |
|---|---|---|
| Genetics | | |
| Alcoholism among 1st or 2nd degree relatives | | |
| Male gender | | |
| Self/Individual/Personal | | |
| Abuse | Antisocial behavior | Parental rejection |
| Learning disorders | | |
| Early onset of drug use | Aggressive temperament | Lack of self control |
| Effects of drugs | | |
| Early sexual activity | Depression | Low self-esteem |
| Body modification (as cutting) | | |
| Attention deficit disorders | Poor self image | Euphoric/mood altering |
| Family | | |
| Dysfunctional family dynamics | | Parental conflict, divorce, separation |
| Permissiveness | | Poor supervision, lack of supervision |
| Authoritarianism | | Poor parental role modeling |
| Community/Environmental/Societal | | |
| Easy availability of drugs and alcohol sanction | | Cultural and religious |
| Acceptance of drug use behavior | | Unemployment |
| Poor general quality of life in the neighborhood | | Low religiosity |
| Media influence and alcohol in certain ethnic groups | | Increased use of drugs |
| Criminal activities in neighborhood | | |
| Peer Group Influence | | |
| Drug using peers | | Curiosity |
| Rebellion | | Desire to belong |
| Rites of passage of puberty | | Independence |
| Risk-taking behavior | | Early tobacco use |
| School/Academic | | |
| Poor school performance | | |
| Poor school environment | | |
| Truancy | | |

[a] Modified with permission: Patel DR, Greydanus DE. 1999. Substance abuse: a pediatric concern. *Indian J. Pediatr.* 66:557–67.

**Table 13.7** Nonspecific indicators of substance abuse.[a]

| Physical | Academic | Behavioral and psychological |
|---|---|---|
| Unexplained weight loss | Deterioration of short-term memory | Risk-taking behavior |
| Hypertension | Poor judgement | Mood swings |
| Red eyes | Falling grades | Depression, withdrawal |
| Nasal irritation | Frequent absence | Panic reaction |
| Frequent "colds" or "allergies" | Truancy | Acute psychosis |
| Hoarseness | Conflicts with teachers | Paranoia |
| Chronic cough | Suspension | Lying |
| Hemoptysis | Expulsion | Stealing |
| Chest pain | | Promiscuity |
| Wheezing | | Conflicts with authorities and family members |
| Frequent unexplained injuries | | Runaway behavior |
| Needle tracks | | Altered sleep pattern |
| Blank stares into space | | Altered appetite |
| Scratch marks | | Poor hygiene |
| Tattoos | | Loss of interest in extracurricular activities |
| Excessive acne | | Drug using peers |
| Testicular atrophy | | Preferences for dress, music, movies identifying with drug – using culture |
| Malaise | | Drug paraphernalia |

[a] Used with permission: Patel DR, Greydanus DE. 1999. Substance abuse: a pediatric concern. *Indian J. Pediatr.*, 66:557–67.

prevalence that is over 80%; this is even higher for the same-aged youth who are school drop-outs. Binge drinking (5 or more alcoholic drinks in males, versus 4 or more in females) is reported in one in every six 14-year-olds, rising to 1 in 3 for 17- to 18-year-olds. Approximately 50% of youth killed in motor vehicle accidents or who commit suicide consume alcohol before their deaths. Current research notes over 50 defined chromosomal regions that may be involved in alcohol addiction.

Alcohol is a CNS depressant leading to rapid euphoria, but later psychological dependence, tolerance, and physiologic dependence in alcoholics.

There can be low-risk use that can lead to such unhealthy patterns as risky use, problem drinking, harmful use, alcohol abuse, and even alcoholism. Alcohol abuse disorder is diagnosed by obtaining a history of excessive alcohol consumption, and not by using a single positive drug test. The abuse of alcohol can lead to anemia along with increase in various laboratory levels, such as liver enzymes, alkaline phosphatase, bilirubin, and uric acid. Acute intoxication can lead to respiratory depression, coma, and even death. Medical complications of excessive alcohol use include incoordination with falls and head injuries, gastritis, pancreatitis, toxic psychosis, and worsening of medical disorders (as diabetes mellitus or epilepsy). The *alcohol withdrawal syndrome* includes tremors, seizures, hallucinations, and delirium tremens. The fetal alcohol syndrome is a well known consequence of alcohol consumption during pregnancy.

## Management of alcohol abuse

A number of screening instruments are available for alcohol abuse, including the CAGE, AUDIT, POSIT, RAFFT, and CRAFFT. Youth should be educated about the dangers of excessive alcohol use. Intensive counseling in a substance abuse program can be of considerable benefit to youth having alcohol abuse disorder; treatment of comorbid conditions, such as depression, is also important. Self-help groups (*Alcohol Anonymous* [AA] and *Alateen* [for adolescents]), and *Adult Children of Alcoholics* can be very helpful to those struggling with alcohol dependence and to those needing information.

Treatment of *acute alcohol consumption* includes gastric emptying, intravenous fluids along with glucose, respiratory support, and, if necessary, dialysis. A number of medications have been used to treat *alcohol withdrawal syndrome*, as noted in Table 13.8; benzodiazepines are sedation-inducing drugs and include diazepam, chlordiazepoxide, and lorazepam that are given every 1–2 hours until withdrawal symptoms cease.

Table 13.9 lists drugs approved for treatment of adults with *alcohol dependence* in the USA; there are no FDA-approved medications for adolescents. The US FDA approved of the use of disulfiram for the management of adult alcohol dependence nearly a half century ago. In 1994, the FDA approved naltrexone (an opioid-receptor antagonist) for management of adult alcohol dependence, followed in 2004 by acamprosate. Other drugs (Table 13.9) have been used in adults with alcohol dependence but are not FDA approved and not discussed here.

**Table 13.8** Medications for management of alcohol withdrawal syndrome.

- Lorazepam (2–4 mg)
- Chlordiazepoxide (50–100 mg)
- Diazepam (10–20 mg)
- Clorazepate
- Various antipsychotics

**Table 13.9** Drugs for management of adults with alcohol dependence.

Approved
   Disulfiram
   Naltrexone
   Acamprosate
Used but not officially approved (Off-label)
   Buspirone
   Calcium carbimide
   Carbamazepine
   Nalmefene (opioid antagonist)
   Ondansetron
   Selective serotonin reuptake inhibitors (e.g. fluoxetine, sertraline)
   Tiapride
   Topiramate (anticonvulsant)
   Tricyclic antidepressants

Table 13.10 reviews the mechanism, side effects, and dosages of the three medications listed; liver function tests (aminotransferase levels) must be monitored when taking disulfiram or naltrexone.

*Drug Interactions*
- Disulfiram may interfere with the metabolism of certain medications, such as phenytoin (causing phenytoin intoxication), oral anticoagulants (prolonged prothrombin time), and isoniazid (mental status changes, unsteady gait).
- Naltrexone blocks opioid effects and can precipitate an acute opioid withdrawal syndrome if given to someone taking opioids; the individual must be off opioids for at least 7–10 days before taking naltrexone. Combining naltrexone with acamprosate increases serum acamprosate levels, but adverse reactions are not seen. Naltrexone is hepatotoxic at higher than recommended levels.

**Table 13.10** FDA medications approved for adult alcohol dependence.

| Agent | Mechanism | Adverse effects | Dosage |
|---|---|---|---|
| Disulfiram (Antabuse, others) | Interferes with alcohol metabolism by inhibition of acetaldehyde dehydrogenase; if even a small amount of alcohol is consumed while on disulfiram, the concentration of acetaldehyde can be 5 to 10 times higher than if the alcohol is consumed without the disulfiram; this is called the disulfiram-alcohol reaction. Tolerance does not develop; increased sensitivity to disulfiram may develop over time. | Drinking alcohol while on disulfiram leads to flushing, headache, nausea, emesis, dyspnea, and confusion. Side effects apart from alcohol ingestion: sleepiness, dermatitis, headache, garlicky taste in mouth; can be hepatotoxic with rare idiosyncratic fulminant hepatitis with death (**Must monitor liver function tests while on this medication**). Also rare: peripheral neuropathy, optic neuritis, polyneuritis, cardiac arrhythmias, and psychosis. Avoid in renal failure; teratogenic; can block tetrahydrocannabinol (THC) metabolism to increase psychoactive effects of marijuana. The patient must avoid alcohol in cough medications, foods, and others. | 125–500 mg a day for the first one to two weeks; maintenance dose is 250 mg (125 to 500 mg). Not approved for those under 18 years of age. |
| Oral naltrexone (ReVia; Depade) FDA approval: 1994 | Inhibits reward effects of alcohol and thus decreases desire for alcohol; blocks effects of opioids (including | Nausea, emesis, dry mouth, insomnia, lethargy, anxiety, dyspepsia, dizziness, headache, increased liver enzymes, eosinophilia. Has black box warning about | **Oral form:** start with 12.5–25 mg a day and maintain on 50 mg a day. |

| | | | |
|---|---|---|---|
| IM (intramuscular) naltrexone (Vivitrol) FDA approval: 2006 | anti-diarrheas and anti-tussives). | hepatotoxic potential seen at or over 5 times recommended dose; **Monitor liver enzymes (aminotransferase levels);** depression and suicide also seen. Can precipitate acute opioid withdrawal syndrome and not given until 7–10 days after opioid is stopped. | **IM form:** 380 mg (4 ml) once a month (provides 3–4 times greater exposure to naltrexone than oral form; safety and efficacy in those under age 18 not established. |
| Acamprosate calcium (Campral) Used in France and other countries since 1989 and FDA-approved in 2004 | It is a synthetic homotaurine derivative which is similar in structure to gamma-amino-butyric acid (GABA); reduces the desire for alcohol use; activates $\gamma$-aminobutyric acid type A receptors and blocks glutaminergic-N-methyl-D-aspartate receptors: decreases glutamatergic transmission and modulates neuronal hyperexcitability after withdrawal/cessation from alcohol ingestion to encourage abstinence. Efficacy rates are similar to naltrexone; can be used with naltrexone or disulfiram. | Main side effect is diarrhea that is dose-related and transient. Others include suicidal ideation and suicides (attempts and completed), nausea, emesis, headache, abdominal pain, drowsiness, dizziness, flatulence, rash, pruritus; avoid in severe renal failure; teratogenic in animals; does not lead to dependence or abuse. | 666 mg (two 333-mg enteric coated tablets) three times a day with meals, starting as soon as possible after alcohol abstinence occurs; lower doses are used by some clinicians; can be continued with a relapse. Not studied in those under 18 years of age. |

- Acamprosate is a safe medication when added to other medications; serum levels are increased when added to naltrexone, but without known adverse consequences.

## Tobacco

Tobacco is another drug that is legal for adults, widely accepted in the world's societies, despite its well-known severe side-effects (including death), and is abused by millions of youth in the world. A number of tobacco products are available, including cigarettes, cigars, chewing tobacco, bidis (brown, hand-rolled, flavored tobacco, also called beedies), kreteks (clove cigarettes containing tobacco and cloves), and others. Even a few cigarettes can occupy enough nicotine receptors in the brain to lead to the need to continue smoking and eventual addiction. In the USA, 1 in 8 of 13–14-year-olds experiment with tobacco while over half of 17- to 18-year-olds who are in school have a lifetime prevalence for smoking cigarettes (nearly 1 in 5 on a daily basis). Approximately 3000 adolescents in the USA start using tobacco every day replacing the 400 000 adults who die each year from their tobacco habit. Over 90% of smoking adults start their tobacco addiction as adolescents. Increased tobacco smoking has been noted in college students in the USA who begin as "social smokers" and then progress to tobacco addiction.

Complications of tobacco use include addiction, heart disease, emphysema, lung cancer, laryngeal carcinoma, oral cancer (from chewing tobacco), and many other disorders. Adolescents are typically more concerned with the *immediate* effects of tobacco (such as bad breath, nicotine-stained teeth, and cough) than with a recitation of the many long-term complications of tobacco addiction. Effects on the offspring of pregnant mothers smoking during their pregnancy include lower birth weight and increased incidence of attention deficit/hyperactivity disorder. The negative effects of passive smoking are also well-recognized by research.

Nicotine is a highly addictive component in tobacco and is absorbed through various sites, including lungs, skin, gastrointestinal tract, and buccal mucosa. Nicotine is quickly bound to the nicotinic acetylcholine receptors found in many non-cholinergic presynaptic and postsynaptic areas of the brain. Other dangerous chemicals found in tobacco include those listed in Table 13.11.

**Table 13.11** Chemicals in tobacco (partial list).

Nicotine
Tar
Carbon monoxide
Arsenous oxide
Radioactive polonium
Benzopyrene
Hundreds of others

## Management of tobacco abuse

The youth of the world should be clearly taught about the many dangers of tobacco use and abuse. Nations should work together to prevent media encouragement of tobacco use and limit societal acceptance of this drug that kills its victims, always looking for new addicts. Tobacco addiction is a powerful neurological disorder and prevention is often more successful than treatment of the addict. FDA-approved pharmacologic approaches in adults with tobacco addiction include the use of nicotine replacement therapies (multiple forms: patch, inhaler, lozenge, and spray), sustained-release bupropion, and varenicline tartrate; none are FDA approved for use in adolescents and there is little research in adolescents available at this time.

Smoking cessation products available in the USA are listed in Tables 13.12 and 13.13. The use of these nicotine replacement products doubles the success rate (from 15% to about 30%) of the committed addict who wishes to stop smoking; a slightly higher rate may occur if bupropion or varenicline is used. Clinicians should use every opportunity to remind smoking adolescents of the dangers of tobacco, establish a "quit" date, and provide support (smoking cessation counseling) as well as pharmacologic management as accepted. Those who stop smoking may experience weight gain, a problem that may be reduced by use of low-dose naltrexone (50–100 mg a day). Naltrexone is an opiate antagonist that binds to the same CNS receptors as the brain reward system's normal neurotransmitters.

The nicotine patch is used for 2 months and changed every morning; a higher strength patch is used for the first month, and then a lower dose for month 2. The patch is not put over a hairy site, and is applied only while awake if insomnia or vivid dreams are noted. Approximately 50% develop local dermatitis, usually resolved with local hydrocortisone cream

**Table 13.12** Pharmacologic management of tobacco addiction in adults.

Approved (adults)
  Nicotine Replacement Treatment
  Bupropion (Zyban)
  Varenicline tartrate (Chantix)
Some research support
  Clonidine
  Nortriptyline
Used without research support
  Buspirone
  Mecamylamine
  Naltrexone
  Doxepin
  Oral dextrose
  Selective serotonin reuptake inhibitors (SSRIs)

application. The nicotine gum (nicotine polacrilex) has a bitter taste not appreciated by most adolescents. A 4 mg piece is chewed by the youth smoking over 25 cigarettes a day, while the 2 mg piece is used for less than 25 cigarettes a day. Side effects include jaw ache, mouth soreness, dyspepsia, and hiccups (Table 13.13). The gum may augment the nicotine patch to reduce acute nicotine cravings. Contraindications to using nicotine replacement therapy (NRT) include pregnancy and cardiovascular diseases.

The nicotine inhaler mimics the hand-to-mouth actions of the smoker and is the preferred nicotine replacement product of some smokers seeking to quit. It is prescribed for 3 months and then slowly tapered off over 3 months. Adverse effects include dyspepsia, irritation of the mouth as well as the throat, nasal irritation, and cough. The nicotine nasal spray is prescribed at a minimum of 8 doses per day, not to exceed 40 a day, or over 5 inhalations per hour. It is not used for those with asthma, since bronchospasm may occur; other side effects include rhinitis, nasal irritation, sneezing, watery eyes, and coughing.

**Bupropion** and **varenicline** are FDA approved for adults. Approximately 25–40% of tobacco addicts who are motivated to quit are successful with using the antidepressant **bupropion**. This drug seems to reduce the addicts' craving for nicotine and improve the complications of depression as well

**Table 13.13** Pharmacologic product guide: smoking cessation.

| | | | Nicotine Replacement Therapy (NRT) Formulations | | | | | | | |
|---|---|---|---|---|---|---|---|---|---|---|
| | | | Transdermal Preparations[OTC/Rx] | | | | | | | |
| Product | Gum[OTC] Nicorette®a, Generic | Lozenge[OTC] Commit®a | Nicotrol Patch®b | Nicoderm® CQ[a] | Generic Patch formerly Habitrol | Generic Patch (formerly Prostep) | Nasal Spray[Rx] Nicotrol NS®b | Oral Inhaler[Rx] Nicotrol Inhaler®b | Bupropion SR[Rx] Zyban®a, Generic | Varenicline tartrate[Rx] Chantix®b,d |
| | • 2 mg, 4 mg: regular, mint, orange | • 2 mg, 4 mg | • 5 mg, 10 mg, 15 mg (16 hour) | • 7 mg, 14 mg, 21 mg (24 hour) | • 7 mg, 14 mg, 21 mg (24 hour) | • 11 mg, 22 mg (24 hour) | • Metered spray (0.5 mg nicotine/ 50uL) aqueous nicotine | • 10 mg cartridge delivers 4 mg inhaled nicotine vapor | • 150 mg sustained-release tablet | • 0.5 mg, 1 mg tablet |
| Precautions | • Pregnancy<br>• Recent (≤2weeks) myocardial infarction<br>• Serious underlying arrhythmias<br>• Serious or worsening angina pectoris<br>• Temporomandibular joint disease | • Pregnancy<br>• Recent (≤2 weeks) myocardial infarction<br>• Serious underlying arrhythmias<br>• Serious or worsening angina pectoris | • Pregnancy<br>• Recent (≤2 weeks) myocardial infarction<br>• Serious underlying arrhythmias<br>• Serious or worsening angina pectoris | | | | • Same as the transdermal preparations Plus:<br>• Underlying chronic nasal disorders (rhinitis, nasal polyps, sinusitis)<br>• Severe reactive airway disease | • Same as the transdermal preparations Plus:<br>• Underlying reactive airway disease | • Pregnancy<br>• Concomitant therapy with medications known to lower the seizure threshold<br>**Contra-indications:**<br>• Hx of seizure disorder, bulimia, anorexia nervosa, MAOI therapy (previous 14days), abrupt d/c of EtOH at same time | • Pregnancy<br>• No clinically meaningful pharmacokinetic drug interactions<br>• Not studied/ recommended in ages <18 years |

(cont.)

**Table 13.13** (cont.)

Nicotine Replacement Therapy (NRT)^OTC/Rx Formulations

| | Gum^OTC Nicorette®ᵃ, Generic | Lozenge^OTC Commit®ᵃ | Transdermal Preparations^OTC/Rx Nicotrol Patch®ᵇ | Nicoderm® CQᵃ | Generic Patch | Generic Patch | Nasal Spray^Rx Nicotrol NS®ᵇ | Oral Inhaler^Rx Nicotrol Inhaler®ᵇ | Bupropion SR^Rx Zyban®ᵃ, Generic | Varenicline tartrate^Rx Chantix®ᵇ,ᵈ |
|---|---|---|---|---|---|---|---|---|---|---|
| **Product** | • 2 mg, 4 mg; regular, mint, orange | • 2 mg, 4 mg | • 5 mg<br>• 10 mg, 15 mg (16 hour) | • 7 mg<br>• 14 mg, 21 mg, (24 hour) | • (formerly Prostep)<br>• 7 mg, 14 mg, 21 mg (24 hour) | • (formerly Habitrol)<br>• 11 mg, 22 mg (24 hour) | • Metered spray (0.5 mg nicotine/50uL) aqueous nicotine | • 10 mg cartridge delivers 4 mg inhaled nicotine vapor | • 150 mg sustained-release tablet | • 0.5 mg, 1 mg tablet |
| **Dosing** | ≥25 cigarettes/day: 4 mg <25 cigarettes/day: 2 mg **Week 1-6:** 1 piece q 1-2 hours **Week 10-12** 1 piece q 4-8 hours<br>• Chew each piece slowly.<br>• Park between cheek and gum when peppery, minty, or citrus taste or tingling sensation appears (~15-30 chews).<br>• Resume chewing when taste or tingle fades.<br>• Repeat chew/park steps until most of the nicotine is gone (taste or tingle does not return; generally 30 min).<br>• Park in different areas of mouth. | 1ˢᵗ cigarette ≤30 minutes after waking up: 4 mg 1ˢᵗ cigarette >30 minutes after waking up: 2 mg **Week 1-6:** 1 lozenge q 1-2 hours **Week 10-12** 1 lozenge q 4-8 hours<br>• Allow lozenge to dissolve slowly (20-30 minutes).<br>• Nicotine release may cause a warm, tingling sensation.<br>• Do not chew or swallow the lozenge. | ≥10 cigarettes/day: 15 mg/d × 6 weeks 10 mg/d × 2 weeks 5 mg/d × 2 weeks ≤10 cigarettes/day **Week 7-9:** NOT recommended<br>• Remove before bedtime<br>• Nicotine released over 16 hours<br>• **Duration:** 10 weeks | ≥10 cigarettes/day: 21 mg/d × 6 weeks 14 mg/d × 2 weeks 7 mg/d × 2 weeks ≤10 cigarettes/day 14 mg/d × 6 weeks 7 mg/d × 2 weeks<br>• May wear patch for 16 hours (remove if patient experiences sleep disturbances.)<br>• **Duration:** 8-10 weeks. | >10 cigarettes/day 21 mg/d × 6 weeks 14 mg/d × 2 weeks 7 mg/d × 2 weeks ≤10 cigarettes/day 14 mg/d × 6 weeks 7 mg/d × 2 weeks<br>• May wear patch for 16 hours (remove if patient experiences sleep disturbances.)<br>• **Duration:** 8-10 weeks | >15 cigarettes/day 22 mg/d × 6 weeks ≤15 cigarettes/day 11 mg/d × 6 weeks<br>• May wear patch for 16 hours (remove if patient experiences sleep disturbances.)<br>• No dose tapering<br>• **Duration:** 6 weeks | 1-2 doses/hour (8-40 doses/day) One dose = 2 sprays (one in each nostril); each spray delivers 0.5 mg of nicotine to the nasal mucosa.<br>• Patients should not sniff, swallow, or inhale through the nose as the spray is administered<br>• For best results, initially use at least 8 doses/d<br>• DO NOT exceed 5 doses/hour or 40 doses/day<br>• Gradually decrease usage over 3-6 months | 6-16 cartridges/day; individualize dosing<br>• Initially, use at least 6 cartridges/day<br>• Best effects with continuous puffing for 20 minutes<br>• Nicotine in cartridge is depleted after 20 minutes of active puffing<br>• Pt should inhale deeply into back of throat or puff in short breaths.<br>• DO NOT inhale into lungs like a cigarette, "puff" as if lighting a pipe. | 150 mg PO q AM × 3 days, then increase to 150 mg PO BID<br>• Treatment should be initiated while patient is still smoking<br>• Set quit date 1-2 weeks after initiation<br>• DO NOT exceed 300 mg/d<br>• Allow at least 8 hours between doses<br>• Avoid bedtime dosing to minimize insomnia<br>• Dose tapering is NOT necessary<br>• Can be used safely with NRT | Recommended 1-week titration: **Days 1-3:** 0.5 mg tablet daily **Days 4-7:** 0.5 mg tablet BID (AM and HS) **Days 8-:** 1 mg tablet BID (AM and HS)<br>• Set quit date<br>• Start Chantix one week before quit date<br>• Take after eating and with a full glass of water<br>• Nausea associated with Chantix is dose related; if persistent and troubling, consider dose reduction |

| | | | | | | | | | |
|---|---|---|---|---|---|---|---|---|---|
| | • No food or beverages 15 minutes before or during use • Max: 20/day • Duration: up to 12 weeks | • Rotate the lozenge to different areas of the mouth • No food or beverages 15 minutes before or during use. • Max: 30 pieces/day • Duration: up to 12 weeks | • Duration: 6 weeks | | | • Open cartridge retains potency for 24 hours • Duration: Up to 6 months | • Duration: 8–12 weeks, maintenance up to 6 months | • Duration: 12 weeks; if successful after 12 weeks, an additional 12 weeks is recommended for increased likelihood of long-term abstinence | |
| **Adverse Events** | • Mouth/jaw soreness • Hiccups • Dyspepsia • Hypersalivation • Effects associated with incorrect chewing technique: -Lightheadedness -Nausea/vomiting -Throat and mouth irritation | • Nausea • Hiccups • Cough • Heartburn • Headache • Flatulence • Insomnia | • Local skin reactions -Erythema -Pruritis -Burning • Headache | • Local skin reactions (erythema, pruritis, burning) • Headache • Sleep disturbances (insomnia) or abnormal dreams associated with nocturnal nicotine absorption | | • Nasal and/or throat irritation (hot, peppery, or burning sensation) • Rhinitis • Tearing • Sneezing • Cough • Headache | • Mouth and/or throat irritation • Unpleasant taste • Cough • Rhinitis • Dyspepsia • Hiccups • Headache | • Insomnia • Dry mouth • Nervousness/difficulty concentrating • Rash • Constipation • Seizures (risk is 1/1000) | • Dose dependent nausea (most common) • Sleep disturbance • Constipation • Flatulence • Vomiting |
| **Advantages** | • Might satisfy oral cravings • May delay weight gain • Pt can titrate therapy to manage withdrawal symptoms • OTC | • Might satisfy oral cravings • May delay weight gain • Pt can titrate therapy to manage withdrawal symptoms • OTC | • Provides consistent nicotine levels over 16 hours • Easy to use and conceal • Fewer compliance issues are associated with the patch • OTC | • Provides consistent nicotine levels over 24 hours • Easy to use and conceal • Fewer compliance issues are associated with the patch • OTC | • Provides consistent nicotine levels over 24 hours • Involves a 1-step process • Easy to use and conceal • Fewer compliance issues associated with the patch • OTC or Rx | • Patients can easily titrate therapy to rapidly manage withdrawal symptoms | • Patients can easily titrate therapy to rapidly manage withdrawal symptoms • The inhaler mimics hand-to-mouth ritual of smoking | • Bupropion can be used with NRT • Bupropion may be beneficial in patients with depression | • Chantix works by two mechanisms: 1)Provides nicotine effects to reduce withdrawal symptoms 2)Blocks the nicotine effects from smoking • No clinically meaningful drug interactions |

**Table 13.13** (cont.)

Nicotine Replacement Therapy (NRT) Formulations

| | Gum^OTC Nicorette®ᵃ, Generic | Lozenge^OTC Commit®ᵃ | Transdermal Preparations^OTC/Rx | | | | Nasal Spray^Rx Nicotrol NS®ᵇ | Oral Inhaler^Rx Nicotrol Inhaler®ᵇ | Bupropion SR^Rx Zyban®ᵃ, Generic | Varenicline tartrate^Rx Chantix®ᵇ,ᵈ |
| | | | Nicotrol Patch®ᵇ | Nicoderm® CQᵃ | Generic Patch | Generic Patch | | | | |
|---|---|---|---|---|---|---|---|---|---|---|
| Product | • 2 mg, 4 mg regular, mint, orange | • 2 mg, 4 mg | • 5 mg, 10 mg, 15 mg (16 hour) | • 7 mg, 14 mg, 21 mg, (24 hour) | • formerly Habitrol • 7 mg, 14 mg, 21 mg (24 hour) | • (formerly Prostep) • 11 mg, 22 mg (24 hour) | • Metered spray (0.5 mg nicotine/ 50uL) aqueous nicotine | • 10 mg cartridge delivers 4 mg inhaled nicotine vapor | • 150 mg sustained-release tablet | • 0.5 mg, 1 mg tablet |
| Disadvantages | • Gum chewing may not be socially acceptable • Difficult to use with dentures • Pt must use proper chewing technique to minimize adverse effects | • Gastrointestinal side effects might be bothersome | • Pts cannot titrate the dose • Allergic reactions to the adhesive might occur • 16-hour patch may lead to early morning cravings • Pts with dermatologic conditions should NOT use the patch | • Pts cannot titrate the dose • Allergic reactions to the adhesive might occur • Pts with dermatologic conditions should NOT use the patch | | | • Nasal/throat irritation may be bothersome • Dependence can result • Pts must wait 5 minutes before driving or operating heavy machinery • Pts with chronic nasal disorders or severe reactive airway disease should NOT use the spray | • Initial throat or mouth irritation can be bothersome • Cartridges should not be stored in very warm conditions or used in very cold conditions • Pts with underlying bronchospastic disease must use with caution | • Seizure risk is increased • Pts with anorexia or bulimia nervosa should not use Bupropion • Pts with a hx of seizures or those taking meds that can lower the seizure threshold should NOT take Bupropion | • Not studied in ages <18 • Not studied in combination with NRT • Nausea associated with higher doses may be bothersome |
| Cost/day^c | 2 mg: $3.92 (9 pieces) 4 mg: $3.92 (9 pieces) | 2 mg: $5.62 (9 pieces) 4 mg: $5.62 (9 pieces) | $3.57 | $3.49–$3.79 | $2.35–$2.70 | $2.20–$2.25 | $3.40 for 10 doses | $11.00 for 6 cartridges | $3.00 | |

Resources: Chart constructed by Courtney Clark, PharmD Candidate

ᵃ Marketed by GlaxoSmithKline. May 2006

ᵇ Marketed by Pfizer.

ᶜ Product pricing based on Walmart in store price quotes. Kalamazoo, MI. Obtained on May 17, 2006.

ᵈ *Chantix prescribing information.* May 2006; Pfizer, Inc. New York, NY. Viewed May 15, 2006. <http://www.pfizer.com/pfizer/download/uspi_chantix.pdf>

ᵉ The regents of the University of California San Francisco, University of Southern California, and Western University of Health Sciences.

as weight gain associated with nicotine cessation. It inhibits reuptake of dopamine and norepinephrine.

In the USA, sustained-release bupropion (bupropion SR), as a treatment for tobacco addiction, is prescribed at an oral dose of 150 mg a day for three days, and then 150 mg twice daily (Table 13.13). It should not be prescribed over 300 mg a day and not taken less than 8 hours apart to reduce the risk of seizures. Its mechanism of action for treatment of tobacco addiction is unknown, but probably involves its noradrenergic and/or dopaminergic actions (see Chapter 6). Bupropion is contraindicated in those with a brain tumor, epilepsy, an eating disorder, or taking medications that lower seizure threshold; it is also contraindicated in patients taking monoamine oxidase inhibitors. Side effects of bupropion include insomnia (40%), dry mouth (10%), headaches, tremors, and dermatological reactions. Selective serotonin reuptake inhibitors have not proven to be effective in smoking cessation. Clonidine and nortriptyline have some positive effects but have a greater side effect profile than noted with bupropion. It is not FDA approved for those under 18 years of age (see Chapter 6).

A newer medication that is FDA approved for use in adults with nicotine addiction is **varenicline tartrate**, an $\alpha 4 \beta 2$ nicotinic acetylcholine receptor partial agonist that binds with more affinity than nicotine to $\alpha 4 \beta 2$ nicotinic acetylcholine receptors; it prevents nicotine from binding and may be more effective than bupropion. The most common adverse effect was nausea that tends to become less severe with continued use. Other side effects include agitation, suicidality, abnormal dreams, constipation, emesis, flatulence, and xerostomia. Mild physical dependence can develop, though overt abuse and addiction are not noted. Weight gain is not reported by users of this medication. Dosing in adults is started at 0.5 mg once a day for 3 days, then twice a day for 4–7 days. It is then increased to 1 mg twice a day for 3 months or longer if necessary.

*Drug interactions*

- Bupropion may interfere with medications metabolized by the CYP2D6 isoenzyme (including SSRIs, TCAs, beta-blockers, antipsychotics, anti-arrhythmics, others; see Chapter 6). It may also interact with drugs metabolized by the CYP2B6 isoenzyme (e.g. cyclophosphamide). Some drugs induce bupropion metabolism (such as phenytoin, phenobarbital, carbamazepine); others (e.g. cimetidine) may inhibit bupropion metabolism. Drug interactions may occur between bupropion and drugs that are metabolized by the CYP2D6 isoenzyme, including MAO inhibitors, amantadine, levodopa, and others. Adding bupropion SR to medications that lower seizure threshold (such as prednisone, antidepressants, antipsychotics, others) should be done only with extreme caution.

- Varenicline has minimal effects on the cytochrome P450 system. Cimetidine ($H_2$ antagonist) decreases varenicline renal clearance and increases its levels in the serum; using both varenicline and transdermal nicotine increases adverse effects, such as nausea, emesis, dizziness, headache, fatigue, and dyspepsia.

Finally, the nicotine vaccine is a new treatment option, now being developed, that increases nicotine antibodies that bind to nicotine and reduce or prevent nicotine distribution in the brain. Research notes that those who receive the vaccine do not develop nicotine withdrawal, such as nicotine craving, or irritability. Side-effects to the vaccine include cough, headache, muscle pain, upper respiratory tract infections, and inflammation of the nose and throat.

## Marijuana

Marijuana (also called "pot," "hash," "weed," "grass," and many other names) is a popular illegal drug of abuse that involves millions of the world's youth. Approximately three-quarters of the illegal drug use in the USA is pot, and nearly 50% of 17–18-year-old youth in school have a lifetime use. In 2005, approximately 35% of American 12th graders reported a past-year use of marijuana. This drug comes from the *Cannabis sativa* plant and its active chemical is *delta-9-tetrahydrocannabinol* or *THC*. The potency of this drug varies considerably, from 1% to 25%, depending on where it is grown.

It is usually smoked, though it can be consumed orally in food and taken orally as a tablet to manage emesis (as noted in chemotherapy for cancer patients), relieve pain in cancer or multiple sclerosis patients, improve muscle spasm in multiple sclerosis patients, or manage glaucoma. The usual pot "joint" (cigarette) contains approximately 20 mg of THC made from a gram of marijuana buds and leaves. Sometimes a "*blunt*" is smoked, made from a hollowed cigar filled with pot. Marijuana users add the pot to other drugs, such as phencyclidine. It may be dipped in formaldehyde or other organic solvents, dried, and then smoked.

**Table 13.14** Potential adverse effects of marijuana.

Psychological addiction
Withdrawal syndrome
Psychological dependency and tolerance (with heavy use)
Flu-like reaction (after stopping this drug after 24 to 60 hours, lasting up to 2 weeks)
Persistent insomnia (may be helped with trazodone)
Reduced memory spans
Reduced reflexes
Impaired memory spans
Altered perceptions of time
Confusion
Impairment of cognition
Amotivational syndrome (lose interest in school or work success)
Psychological reactions: fear, depression, anxiety, violent behavior, hallucinations
Precipitate overt depression or psychosis
Cough
Bronchitis
Bronchospasm
Amenorrhea
Reduced sperm count
Immunologic dysfunction

Marijuana is a popular drug of abuse because it is easily obtained around the world and produces potent euphoria that starts in minutes and can last for hours. Though considered by addicts and the media (movies, television talk show hosts, and others) to be a harmless drug, marijuana is a dangerous drug of abuse with many potential side effects, as listed in Table 13.14. Pot use can interfere with daily life at school, work, and the home. Its use, often in combination with alcohol, leads to many motor vehicle accidents because drivers are inattentive and have slower reaction times. Some drugs (such as amphetamines and cocaine) enhance the stimulatory effects of marijuana while other drugs (such as alcohol or diazepam) worsen the sedative effects of pot. It is a dangerous drug of abuse and clinicians caring for adolescents should educate their patients to this concept. Convincing a chronic pot addict to stop this drug is very difficult. There are no known psychopharmacologic agents shown to help the chronic pot user stop using this drug.

**Table 13.15** Amphetamine adverse reactions.

Exhaustion
Insomnia
Hyperactivity
Anorexia
Anxiety
Weight loss
Intravenous use complications (HIV/AIDS, endocarditis, hepatitis, and other infections)
Tolerance
Personality changes
Hyperhidrosis
Hypertension
Mydriasis
Overdose (hyperthermia, hypertension, cardiac arrhythmias, seizures, and death)
Personality changes
Psychotic experiences
Tachycardia
Withdrawal syndrome (severe apathy, depression, and hypersomnia)

# ■ Amphetamines

Amphetamine (also called *meth, speed, chalk,* and others) is a well-known stimulant of the central nervous system with many potential side effects, as noted in Table 13.15. It is taken to become euphoric, reduce the sense of fatigue, cause weight loss, reduce attention span problems, and/or improve sports performance. Amphetamines are taken in many forms: orally, subcutaneously, or intravenously. Approximately 15% of American 17- to 18-year-olds in school have a lifetime prevalence of amphetamine use. Overdose management involves use of a cooling blanket for hyperthermia, control of hypertension as well as arrhythmias with medications, and use of medications (haloperidol or droperidol) for delusions or agitation. Other medications used for agitation include diazepam or lorazepam. Health care providers prescribing amphetamines for attention deficit/hyperactivity disorder (ADHD) should be aware of the potential for abuse by these patients (see Chapter 5), or diversion to others.

## Methamphetamine

This illegal drug has become a favorite stimulant of adolescents throughout the world. It has many names (*meth, ice, fire, glass, crystal,* and others) and

**Table 13.16** Potential side effects of methamphetamine.

Aggressiveness and violent behavior
Anxiety
Cardiac damage, cardiovascular collapse, and death
Confusion
Convulsions
Hypertension
Irritability
Insomnia
Intravenous complications: overdose, HIV/AIDS, endocarditis, others
Memory loss
Tremors
Paranoia and psychotic behavior

is an N-methyl homolog of amphetamine. Methamphetamine is a highly addictive chemical easily prepared by clandestine laboratories using cheap ingredients (as over-the-counter cold medications) and sold throughout the world as a white powder (odorless and bitter-tasting) or clear crystals. It is abused as a pill or powder taken orally, inhaled (smoked), or injected. It is highly lipophilic and easily crosses the blood–brain barrier leading to a rapid, potent euphoria lasting a matter of minutes, but can set up a lifetime quest for more of this drug. The addict notes increased wakefulness, reduced sleep requirements, and hyperactivity. Vital signs are increased, with increased temperature, pulse, respirations, and blood pressure. Speech patterns are described as "excited" and drug-induced brain dopamine release affects mood and body movements.

As brain cells containing dopamine and serotonin are damaged, problems arise, including depression, reduced thinking ability, and even a parkinsonian-like movement disorder. Table 13.16 lists potential adverse effects of methamphetamine abuse. Management of this powerfully addictive drug is very difficult and depends on a firm resolve on the addict's part to recover. There is no pharmaceutical chemical that is effective in treating methamphetamine addiction. The beta-blockers are used to manage cardiac arrhythmias noted in acute methamphetamine intoxication, while a benzodiazepine (such as lorazepam or others) is used to manage irritability or agitation; an antipsychotic medication is used for psychotic symptoms, but CYP2D6 inhibitors (such as haloperidol) are avoided, since they may increase serum methamphetamine levels. Patients with methamphetamine addiction should be provided with intense psychological therapies, perhaps supplemented with an antidepressant (such as bupropion).

Research is currently seeking a medication to block the euphoric effects of methamphetamine. The development of such an "antibody" to neutralize this drug is also being sought for other drug addictions, including cocaine, heroin, and others. A current drug under investigation to reduce methamphetamine addiction is GVG (gamma-vinyl GABA). Research has noted that nicotine and donepezil (an anti-Alzheimer drug) can reduce the craving for methamphetamine; both drugs stimulate nicotinic acetylcholine receptors which are part of the brain's reward system.

## ■ Cocaine

Cocaine is a central nervous system stimulant that is known as one of the most addictive and dangerous drugs of abuse in the world. It is made from *Erythroxylon coca*, a plant found in South America. Profound euphoria can be obtained after taking cocaine in various ways, including swallowing, chewing (coca leaves), inhalation, smoking, intranasally, and intravenously. It was originally produced as a crystalline powder; however, *crack* cocaine is now popular in a smoking form, either by itself or added to tobacco or marijuana. Various other chemicals can be added, such as quinine or mannitol. Approximately 1 in 4 Americans try cocaine before reaching their 30th birthday, and 17- to 18-year-olds who are in school report a nearly 8% lifetime use record for the drug.

The potent euphoria lasts up to 10 minutes if the cocaine is smoked and up to 30 minutes with intravenous use. Once the cocaine high wears off, profound irritability and fatigue develops. Abuse of cocaine leads to severe addiction (psychological and physiological) and tolerance. Cocaine addicts have lower concentrations of CNS $D_2$ dopamine receptors than non-cocaine users. Addicts often add various chemicals such as alcohol or heroin to the cocaine to augment the drug experience; however, this also increases the risk for sudden death. Table 13.17 provides a list of some of the potential complications of cocaine addiction.

### Management of cocaine addiction

Treatment of cocaine abuse is a difficult problem and as with many types of substance abuse disorders, prevention is preferable to management of overt addiction. There are no medications to effectively treat cocaine

**Table 13.17** Adverse effects of cocaine.

Anxiety
Cardiac complications
  Angina pectoris
  Myocardial infarction
  Ventricular arrhythmia
  Sudden death
Confusion
Fontal lobe infarction
Hyperpyrexia, tachycardia, and hypertension
Irritability and restlessness,
Intravenous needle complications (including hepatitis B, HIV/AIDS, endocarditis)
Nasal septum infection and perforation
Paranoia (seen with smoking cocaine)
Peripheral blood vessel constriction
Pregnancy complications
  Increased premature delivery
  Abruption (bleeding between placenta and uterine wall)
  Adverse neurodevelopmental sequelae in infants
  Vascular spasm-induced limb reduction anomalies and strokes
Pupillary dilation
Seizures

addiction. Short-acting beta-blockers and direct vasodilators are helpful with cocaine-related tachycardia and hypertension; some clinicians do not use beta-blockers because of risk of reduced coronary perfusion and increased myocardial infarction in acute cocaine intoxication. Benzodiazepines induce sedation and can help manage seizure activity, while the risk of cerebrovascular accidents may be reduced with the use of a calcium channel blocker (dihydropyrimidine-type). Healthcare professionals should avoid long-acting vasodilators, since cocaine intoxication does not usually last long. Naloxone, useful for opioid addiction, is not helpful for cocaine abuse.

Cocaine addicts who also have ADHD note that stimulants like *methylphenidate* (MPH) calms them down and may allow less cocaine use. Cocaine addicts who also have ADHD may benefit from 40–60 mg of sustained-release MPH in reducing pathological craving for cocaine. Research is currently seeking drugs to block the effects of cocaine – and prevent its euphoric effect – on multiple brain sites. Drugs such as dopamine $D_3$ receptor agonists ($D_3$ agonists) may neutralize cocaine in the blood and

**Table 13.18** Narcotic opiates.

Heroin
Codeine
Oxycodone
Fentanyl
Propoxyphene
Meperidine
Methadone
Morphine
Pentazocine
Hydrocodone

help with cocaine addiction, overdose, and drug-induced seizure activity. One example currently being researched is called TA-CD; another is GVG (gamma-vinyl GABA). Topiramate (an anticonvulsant) has been shown in research trials to help cocaine addicts stay off cocaine; it can exacerbate cocaine withdrawal and is not used until the addict has been off cocaine for 3 days or more. Topiramate has been used to prevent relapse in those with alcohol, opiate, and cocaine addiction; it may help with nicotine addiction as well. Drugs used to treat alcohol abuse may be of help to cocaine addicts who also abuse alcohol; these drugs include disulfiram and naltrexone (see Table 13.10).

## ■ Opioids

Table 13.18 lists various opiate narcotics that are abused by youth as well as adults. Comments in this section focus on heroin (diacetyl morphine hydrochloride), a powerful addictive drug available around the world, and used as a snuff, intravenously, or subcutaneously. Although it was outlawed in the USA in 1925, approximately 3 million Americans have abused heroin in recent times. The abuse of heroin has doubled in American adolescents since the late 1990s, and abuse of prescription opiates (e.g. oxycodone and hydrocodone) has increased even more. The use of oxycodone among adolescents has increased from 4.0% in 2002 to 5.5% in 2005, while use of hydrocodone has remained high – 9.6% in 2002 and 9.5% in 2005.

A popular method of abuse is to combine heroin with cocaine ("speedball") to blunt the severe sedative effects of heroin. Heroin has many street names, including *China white, smack, junk,* and *Mexican brown.* The adolescent often first snorts this drug and becomes addicted to its powerful

**Table 13.19** Medical complications of heroin abuse.

Physical addiction
Psychological dependence
Withdrawal syndrome
Overdose (respiratory depression, pulmonary edema, death)
Newborn withdrawal syndrome
Amenorrhea
Complications from intravenous use
   Endocarditis (from *Staphylococcus aureus*)
   HIV/AIDS
   Hepatitis B and C
   Osteomyelitis
   Tetanus
False-positive VDRL
Fat necrosis
   Lipodystrophy
Peptic ulcer disease
Pulmonary edema and pneumonia
Respiratory arrest
Others

euphoric effects, leading to eventual smoking and/or intravenous use. A profound physical addiction then results, along with psychological dependence and a connection that is very difficult to break. Medical complications are numerous, as partially outlined in Table 13.19. Tattoos are often used to hide the scars from intravenous heroin use.

## Heroin addiction management

Research notes that addiction, such as that noted with heroin, is a neurobiological condition of the central nervous system involving many opiate receptors. Drugs of abuse block the dopamine transporter in the brain's reward circuits, a process complicated perhaps by reduced numbers of CNS $D_2$ receptors in addicts. These youth need acute detoxification measures followed by intense treatment of the addiction process, often in residential treatment facilities, if available.

Naloxone hydrochloride is an opiate antagonist and is used to manage overdose due to opioids (such as heroin); intravenous (IV) administration is recommended in emergency situations, though it can be given intramuscularly (IM) or subcutaneously (SC) as well. In cases of heroin overdose, it is given at a dose of 0.4–2 mg IV and repeated every 2–3 minutes until improvement in respiratory depression occurs; it is also used to improve sedation and hypotension noted in the overdose. If a total of 10 mg has been given, the overdose may not be due to an opioid. In children, a trial IV dose of 0.01 mg/kg body weight is given followed by an IV dose of 0.1 mg/kg body weight if necessary. A relapse of the heroin overdose symptoms may occur over the next 24 hours as the naloxone is metabolized. Naloxone can lead to hypotension, acute opioid withdrawal syndrome, cardiac arrhythmias, emesis, and other adverse effects. Management of the pregnant mother who is on heroin and is delivering includes the use of naloxone for the mother and the neonate as necessary; IV administration is recommended for the neonate.

Lofexidine hydrochloride is an $\alpha_2$ adrenergic agonist used in the UK and other countries to treat opiate withdrawal over a 5–10 day period; side effects include hypotension, sedation, and dry mucous membranes. It is started at 0.2 mg twice daily, and increased by 0.2–0.4 mg to a maximum daily dose of 2.4 mg; it is gradually withdrawn over 2–4 days.

*Heroin dependence management* Intensive behavioral therapy is necessary to help heroin addicts recover and community programs like Narcotics Anonymous (NA) are helpful as well. Youth who are addicted to heroin or other narcotic opiates should be under the care of an addiction specialist well trained in these various antinarcotic medications. Behavioral interventions are a major part of treatment for adolescents and adults addicted to heroin and other opiates.

A number of medications are used to help blunt the profound euphoric effects of heroin by serving as opioid replacement therapy; these medications include naltrexone, methadone hydrochloride, LAAM (levo-alpha-acetylmethadol or levomethadyl acetate), and buprenorphine hydrochloride. Other medications used to help with the treatment of opioid addiction include alpha$_2$-adrenergic agonists (e.g. clonidine), antidepressant drugs (such as SSRIs), and anti-anxiety medications (such as buspirone). In a few countries (e.g. the UK), heroin is available as diamorphine and has been prescribed (with a clean needle) for several decades to a select group of those with severe, refractory heroin addiction. Anesthesia-assisted detoxification, using anesthesia for 4–6 hours on day 1 of opiate detoxification, is a method that is not FDA approved and is not supported by research to be an effective detoxification method for opioid addicts.

Naltrexone is an opioid-receptor antagonist that blocks $\mu$-opioid receptors and is used to manage opioid dependence, though more research is needed to establish its actual efficacy in this situation. It is not given until a week or more after the addict is free of opioids; if given sooner, opioid withdrawal symptoms may develop that are sudden and severe. The maintenance dose for naltrexone is 50 mg per day; some start at 12.5 mg, increase to 25 mg and then to 50 mg per day (Table 13.10). Heroin overdose risks seem to be increased for those who stop taking naltrexone for heroin dependence treatment, more so than other medications that are used for sobriety and then stopped.

Methadone is a $\mu$-opioid receptor agonist and has been available for over 40 years (Table 13.20). Use of methadone to treat narcotic addiction has been a controversial treatment since its beginning in the 1960s. In the USA, methadone is reserved for the individual severely addicted to heroin who typically must take naltrexone to prove they are not on heroin when taking the methadone, since naltrexone will precipitate an opiate withdrawal state. In the UK, other European countries, and Australia, methadone is provided to the less severely addicted individual and maintenance is the main goal of its use. In the USA, methadone for the treatment of opiate addiction can only be dispensed through approved treatment facilities.

A search for longer-acting treatment medications led to the current use of buprenorphine and levomethadyl acetate (LAAM). Buprenorphine is a partial opioid receptor agonist given as sublingual tablets and has fewer side effects than does methadone, including being safer in overdose (Table 13.20). It was developed in the 1970s as an injectable pain medication, and can be prescribed by any physician who has taken an 8-hour course in its management so that a patient can get this medication from the trained physician in the office, picked up at a pharmacy, and taken at home. The Drug Addiction Treatment Act of 2000 (DATA 2000) sets up how a physician can qualify to use Schedule III, IV, and V narcotic medications in the USA to manage opioid addiction in facilities other than the methadone clinic. Certification is through the US Substance Abuse and Mental Health Services Administration (SAMHSA). The purpose of this extended use of this medication is to allow the treatment of opioid addiction to be similar to that of other chronic illnesses in which primary care clinicians care for many of

**Table 13.20** FDA-approved medications used for heroin dependence treatment.

| Agent | Mechanism | Adverse effects | Dosage |
|---|---|---|---|
| Methadone (Dolophine, others) | μ-opioid receptor agonist that blocks narcotic effects while avoiding basic narcotic euphoria; can eliminate opiate withdrawal symptoms and lessen need for additional addictive drugs. | Addiction to methadone; worsen other addictions, as cocaine addiction; cardiac arrhythmias (need electrocardiogram monitoring). Patient needs to get a daily dose from highly regulated, government programs in USA. Preferred drug for pregnant heroin addict. | 20–100 mg maintenance (maximum: 400 mg a day); patient takes naltrexone to prove they are not on heroin, since naltrexone can precipitate opiate withdrawal. |
| Buphenorphine (Subutex; other) (sublingual tablets: 2, 8 mg) | Schedule III partial opioid receptor agonist used for detoxification and maintenance treatment of heroin and other narotics. | Opioid withdrawal may develop if buphenorphine is given to someone with recent opioid use. Sedation is a common adverse effect (2/3 of patients); others: nausea, dizziness/ vertigo. Less common: headache, emesis, sweating, miosis, hypotension, hypoventilation. Suboxone: high risk for intense withdrawal symptoms if taking opioids due to the naloxone. Interacts with CYP 3A4 inhibitors (as ketoconazole, erythromycin, HIV protease inhibitors). | Gradual increase of 2–4 mg buprenorphine to daily maintenance of 16 mg (range: 4–24 mg for some); can start with buprenorphine along and then use Suboxone. Can prescribe in the office after taking 8 hours course. Safety below age 16 years not established. |
| Buprenorphine/naloxone (Suboxone) (sublingual tablets: 2/0.5 mg and 8/2 mg) | Developed in the 1970s as an injectable analgesic. Opposes heroin effects and addict has less euphoria with heroin if on this medication. | | |
| Levomethadyl acetate (LAAM; levo-alpha-acetylmethadol; Orlaam). | Synthetic opioid analgesic with actions similar to methadone but longer-acting: 48 to 72 hours. | *Torsades de pointes* (ventricular tachycardia with prolonged QT intervals); avoid with prolonged QT and conditions/drugs that may cause this; monitor with electrocardiograms; high abuse potential and overdose may occur; can also see withdrawal syndrome; other adverse effects: sedation, dizziness, syncope, constipation, dry mouth. Interacts with CYP3A4 inducers (rifampin, phenytoin, phenobarbital); interacts with CYP3A4 inhibitors (ketoconazole, erythromycin, HIV proteinase inhibitors); avoid in pregnancy. | Start with 20 to 40 mg; maximum: 120 mg. Seen in the office 3 times per week; not given to those under age 18 years. See text. |

these addicts in their offices. This model is popular in Europe and is growing in interest in the USA.

Buprenorphine has a longer duration of action (for alternative-day dosing) and induces less analgesic effects than methadone. Opioid withdrawal may develop if buprenorphine is given to someone with recent opioid use. Research suggests it is as effective as methadone for maintenance treatment of heroin addiction and better tolerated than methadone or clonidine for opioid withdrawal. There is also the sublingual combination of buprenorphine/naloxone that was FDA approved in 2002; the naloxone is used to prevent the intravenous administration of the buprenorphine. Patients are typically stabilized on 16 mg of buprenorphine a day and 4 mg of naloxone a day (Table 13.20).

Levomethadyl acetate (LAAM) is a synthetic opioid analgesic and is taken 2–3 times a week instead of the daily administration for methadone. Anecdotal reports of *torsades de pointes* (ventricular tachycardia with prolonged QT intervals) have been linked to LAAM administration, and periodic electrocardiograms are recommended for patients on this medication for opiate dependence treatment. The negative profile of LAAM may result in its ultimate removal from the market.

## ■ Hallucinogenic drugs

The classic hallucinogens include PCP (*phencyclidine*) and LSD (*lysergic acid diethylamide*) that are taken orally to develop a potent distortion of reality with changes in sensory perceptions (involving sound and sight) as well as emotions (involving euphoria and intense fears). Phencyclidine is an arylcyclohexalamine made in illegal laboratories and is taken as a pill, liquid, or powder that can be sprinkled on marijuana cigarettes (joints) to increase the effects of pot. Management of a bad reaction (called a "trip") to PCP ingestion is based on placing the patient in a dark room that is well-padded and giving benzodiazepines (such as diazepam) or haloperidol for severe agitation. Death may occur from a PCP reaction because of hypothermia, seizures, trauma, severe blood pressure changes (hypertension or hypotension), and/or psychotic delirium.

Lysergic acid diethylamide (LSD) is a powerful hallucinogen found in morning glory seeds and rye fungus (*Ergot*). It is an odorless, tasteless, and colorless chemical popular at marathon dances or *raves* where it can be easily given to unsuspecting females. Euphoria or hallucinogenic effects may result from a dose as low as 20 mcg because of the intense increase in serotonin. Other effects include fever, tachycardia, mydriasis, and hypertension. A youth having a "bad trip" or unpleasant "flashback" is usually managed with reassurance; haloperidol is given for severe reactions, such as prolonged agitation.

# ■ MDMA (Ecstasy)

MDMA (3,4 methylenedioxymethamphetamine) is a phenethylamine that resembles both a stimulant (methamphetamine) and a hallucinogen (mescaline). The phenethylamines comprise a group of over 100 hallucinogenic chemicals. A related compound to MDMA is MDEA (3,4-methylenedioxyeth- amphetamine), often called *Eve* on the streets. MDMA is obtained as a crystalline powder, white if pure and red or brown if mixed with impurities; it has many street names, such as *lover's speed, diamonds, clarity, dex,* and many others.

The popularity of *Ecstasy* is based on the profound euphoria it produces along with an energizing effect that has made it a commonly used drug at marathon dances attended by youth around the world. MDMA can enhance sensual awareness and augment psychic or emotional energy. The MDMA high usually lasts 3–6 hours, though sometimes it goes on for several days. It interacts with and can destroy brain serotonergic neurons that regulate memory and thought. MDMA can cause an anxious sense of "well-being," changes in perception, feelings of derealization, and even depersonalization. It is a popular date rape drug (see below).

Table 13.21 lists some of the side effects of MDMA use. Abuse can lead to thinking and memory impairment along with behavioral problems; panic attacks and paranoia may last for several weeks after the drug is stopped. The risk for congenital anomalies is increased if it is taken during pregnancy. It can mask thirst, and death may result from dehydration, hyperthermia, hyponatremia, or cerebral edema. High doses can result in muscle breakdown, malignant hyperthermia and failure of the kidneys and cardiovascular system. Youth with unknown vascular anomalies may develop intracerebral hemorrhage after taking MDMA.

*Date rape drugs* Various designer drugs (such as MDMA) are now made by chemists and introduced to the streets for use by the general public. One byproduct of this production is the development of chemicals that reduce

**Table 13.21** Side effects of MDMA (3, 4 methylene dioxymethamphetamine).

Anxiety, including panic attacks
Confusion and paranoia
Dehydration, sweating, and possible heat stroke
Depression
Fatigue and other sleep dysfunction
Hypertension and increased pulse
Intracerebral hemorrhage
Irreversible CNS damage with memory loss with chronic abuse
Muscle spasms
Organ dysfunction: renal, liver, CNS, muscular
Psychosis
Others

**Table 13.22** Date rape drugs.

Methylenedioxymethamphetamine ("Ecstasy," MDMA)
Methamphetamine
Rohypnol (Flunitrazepam)
Gamma-hydroxybutyrate (GHB)
Gamma-butyryl lactone (GB)
Butanediol (BD)
LSD (lysergic acid diethylamide)
Ketamine (Ketalar)

inhibitions and consciousness. These so called *date rape drugs* (Table 13.22) are given to unsuspecting females by males who then sexually assault the victim; for example, the drug can be added to an alcoholic drink at a party, the two leave the room, and as the female becomes sedated, sexual assault occurs with minimal if any memory of the rape. Date rape drugs are popular at marathon dances and are called *club drugs* or *party drugs*. Some of these chemicals are now briefly reviewed.

## Flunitrazepam

Flunitrazepam is a central nervous system depressant that is a potent benzodiazepine with multiple actions: anticonvulsant, anxiolytic, and sedative. This drug, like the date rape drugs, reduces sexual inhibitions and causes memory loss in which there is no memory for recent events. It is a colorless, odorless, and tasteless chemical that has become a classic date rape pill throughout the world. Flunitrazepam is prescribed in Europe and other areas as a presurgical anesthetic and as medication for the treatment of insomnia. One milligram slipped into a drink will sedate the victim for 8–12 hours. It is also a drug of abuse taken voluntarily to serve as an alternative or added drug to LSD, marijuana, or alcohol. Side effects include sedation, confusion, dizziness, visual disturbances, hypotension, urinary retention, gastrointestinal dysfunction, and others. Flumazenil can be used as an antidote to the toxic effects of flunitrazepam, but can induce cardiac arrhythmias and seizure activity if other drugs are mixed with the flunitrazepam.

## Gamma-hydroxybutyrate (GHB)

Gamma-hydroxybutyrate or GHB (called *liquid ecstasy, Georgia home boy*) is another central nervous system depressant that is used as a date rape drug because it reduces inhibition, enhances euphoria, and is easily slipped into drinks; it is odorless and colorless, though it can have a soapy or salty taste. GBH acts on gamma-amino-butyric acid (GABA) receptors and exerts a powerful addictive effect on its users. GHB works in 10–20 minutes, peaks in 1–2 hours, and is gone in 4 hours; amnesia for recent events is characteristic of this drug. Seizures and death may result from respiratory depression, and may occur when it is combined with alcohol, LSD, heroin, or other drugs. Chronic GHB users can develop intense withdrawal symptoms when stopping this drug.

## Ketamine

Ketamine ("*Special K*") is an injectable anesthetic used for animals that can be abused as a date rape drug. It is a white powder that can be snorted or taken intramuscularly; it can be added to marijuana or tobacco. Ketamine can induce a dream-like or hallucinatory dissociative state in low doses, leading to impaired memory and learning ability, and poor attention span; in higher doses, side effects include hypertension, amnesia, delirium, motor dysfunction, and death from respiratory depression.

## ■ Summary

All clinicians must work with their pediatric and adolescent patients to teach them about the dangers of drug abuse and help them get off the precipitous slide that drugs take our youth down. We must work with various elements of society to reduce this major threat to our children. Prevention of drug abuse is the key to this immense problem and behavioral therapies are the mainstay of drug dependence management. Medications are needed for treatment of various drug withdrawal syndromes and overdoses. Psychopharmacologic management can also be helpful in selected cases, particularly for alcohol dependence, tobacco addiction, and opiate addiction (Tables 13.10, 13.13, and 13.20).

## SELECTED BIBLIOGRAPHY

American Academy of Child and Adolescent Psychiatry. 2005. Practice parameter for the assessment and treatment of children and adolescents with substance use disorders. *J. Am. Acad. Child Adolesc. Psychiatry*, 44:609–21.

American Psychiatric Association. 2000. *Diagnostic and Statistical Manual of Mental Disorders, fourth Edition, Text Revision*. Washington, DC: American Psychiatric Association.

Bukstein OG, Bernet W, Arnold V *et al.* 2005. Practice parameter for the assessment and treatment of children and adolescents with substance abuse disorders. *J. Am. Acad. Child Adolesc. Psychiatry*, 44:609–21.

Cozzolino E, Guglielmino L, Vigezzi P *et al.* 2006. Buprenorphine treatment: a three-year prospective study in opioid-addicted patients of a public out-patient addiction center in Milan. *Am. J. Addict.* 15(3); 246–51.

ESPAD (The European School Survey Project on Alcohol and Other Drugs) Report, 1999.

Fiore MC, Bailey WC, Cohen SJ *et al.* 2000. *Treating Tobacco Use and Dependence. Clinical Practice Guideline*. US Department of Health and Human Services.

Fournier ME, Levy S. 2006. Recent trends in adolescent substance use, primary care screening, and updates in treatment options. *Curr. Opin. Pediatrics*, 352–8.

Galanter M (Ed.) 2006. *Alcohol Problems in Adolescents and Young Adults: Epidemiology, Neurobiology, Prevention, and Treatment*. New York: Springer-Verlag.

Garofalo R, Mustanski BS, McKirnan DJ, *et al.* 2007. Methamphetamine and young men who have sex with men: understanding patterns and correlates of use and the association with HIV-related special risk. *Arch. Pediatr. Adol. Med.*, 161:591–6.

Greydanus DE, Patel DR. 2002. Sports doping in the adolescent: the hope, the hype and the hyperbole. *Pediatr. Clin. N. Am.*, 49(4):829–55.

Greydanus DE, Patel DR. 2003. Substance abuse in adolescents: a complex conundrum for the clinician. *Pediatr. Clin. N. Am.*, 59(5):1179–223.

Greydanus DE, Patel DR. 2005. The adolescent and substance abuse: current concepts. *Curr. Probl. Pediatr. Adolesc. Health Care*, 35(3):1–21.

Greydanus DE, Patel DR. 2006. Adolescents and drug abuse. In *Essentials of Adolescent Medicine*. New York: McGraw-Hill Medical Publishers.

Johnson RE, Chutuape MA, Strain EC *et al.* 2000. A comparison of levomethadyl acetate, buprenorphine, and methadone for opioid dependence. *N. Engl. J. Med.*, 43:1290–7.

Johnston LD, O'Malley PM, Bachman JG. 2006. *The Monitoring the Future Study on Adolescent drug use: Overview of Key Findings. 2005.* National Institutes of Health Publication No. 04–5506. Bethesda, MD: National Institute on Drug Abuse.

Kirchmayer U, Davoli M, Verster A. 2004. *Naltrexone Maintenance Treatment for Opioid Dependence.* The Cochrane Library. Issue 3. Chichester: Johnson and Sons.

Klesges RC, Johnson KC, Somes G. 2006. Varenicline for smoking cessation; definite promise, but no panacea. *J. Am. Med. Assoc.* 296:94–5.

Kranzler HR. 2006. Evidence-based treatments for alcohol dependence: new results and new questions. *J. Am. Med. Assoc.*, 295(17):2075–6.

March LA. 2005. Comparison of pharmacological treatments for opioid-dependent adolescents: a randomized controlled trial. *Arch. Gen. Psychiatry*, 62:1157–64.

Lancaster T, Stead LF. 2000. Individual behavioral counseling for smoking cessation: Cochrane review. In *The Cochrane Library, Issue 2.* Oxford: Update Software Ltd.

Lancaster T, Stead LF. 2000. Self-help interventions for smoking cessation: Cochrane review. In *The Cochrane Library, Issue 2.* Oxford: Update Software Ltd.

National Institute on Drug Abuse. National Institutes of Health: Cigarettes and other nicotine products. www.nida.nih.gov

National Institute on Drug Abuse; United States Department of Health and Human Services. 2000. NIH Publication No. 00–4690.

Patel DR, Greydanus DE. 1999. Substance abuse: A pediatric concern. *Indian J. Pediatr.*, 66: 557–67.

Patel DR, Greydanus DE. 2000. Office interventions for adolescent smokers. *Adolesc. Med.*, 11 (3):1–11.

Roffman RA, Stephens RS (Eds.) 2006. *Cannabis Dependence: Its Nature, Consequences and Treatment.* (International Research Monographs in the Addictions). New York: Cambridge University Press.

Ross S, Hayden F. 2006. *Study Guide to Substance Abuse Treatment: A Companion to the American Psychiatric Publishing Textbook of Substance Abuse Treatment, Third Edition.* Washington, DC: American Psychiatric Publishing.

Schydlower M (Ed.) 2000. *Substance Abuse: A Guide for Health Professionals.* Elk Grove Village, IL: American Academy of Pediatrics.

Schydlower M, Arredondo RM (Eds.) 2006. Substance abuse among adolescents. *Adolesc. Med. Clinics*, 17(2):259–505.

Shiffman S, Johnston JA, Khayrallah M *et al.* 2000. The effect of bupropion on nicotine craving and withdrawal. *Psychopharmacology*, 148:33.

Sofuoglu M, Kosten TR. 2004. Pharmacologic management of relapse prevention in addictive disorder. *Psychiatr. Clin. N. Am.*, 27:624–8.

Sung S, Conry MJ. 2006. Role of buprenorphine in the management of heroin addiction. *Ann. Pharmacother.* 40(3):501–5.

Substance abuse disorders

Upadhyaya H, Deas D, Brady K. 2005. A practical clinical approach to the treatment of nicotine dependence in adolescents. *J. Am. Acad. Adolesc. Psychiatr.* 942–6.

US Department of Health and Human Services. 2000. *Healthy People 2010. Understanding and Improving Health and Objectives for Improving Health. Vols I and II, 2nd Edn.* Washington, DC: US Government Printing Office.

2006. Varenicline (Chantix) for tobacco dependence. *Med. Lett.* 48:66–8.

Williams JF. 2007. Inhalant abuse. *Pediatrics*, 119:1009–17.

Williams SH. 2005. Medications for treating alcohol dependence. *Am. Fam. Phys.*, 72:1775–80.

## Internet

National Institute on Drug Abuse: www.nida.gov/NIDAHome.html

National Clearinghouse on Alcohol and Drug Information: www.health.org

National Institute on Alcohol Abuse and Alcoholism: www.niaaa.nih.gov

http://www.MonitoringTheFuture.org

www.fda.gov/medwatch/safety/2008/safety08.htm#Antiepileptic

# Subject index

Notes, the following abbreviations have been used:
ADHD – attention deficit hyperactivity disorder
ASD – autistic spectrum disorder
DSM-IV-TR – Diagnostic and Statistical Manual of Mental Disorders
SSRIs – selective serotonin reuptake inhibitors

Printed in the United States
by Baker & Taylor Publisher Services